Somatic Intelligence – Volume 7

# You Are the Fulcrum

Using the conscious language of the body to heal

By Suresha Hill, EdS, HSE, DOMTP

Front cover photo courtesy of Frank Cone

Cover designs by Suresha Hill and Tamera Haney

Edited with help from Sharon, James, Loraine, Mark, and Allison

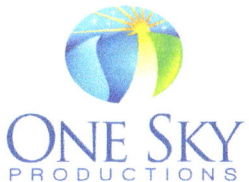

All Rights Reserved © 2020
No portion of this text, except for brief review, may be reproduced, stored in an electronic retrieval system, or transmitted in any form, by any means - electronic, photocopying, recording, or otherwise without the expressed, written permission of the author and publisher: One Sky Productions, P.O. Box 150954
San Rafael, CA 94915

# Table of Contents

| | |
|---|---|
| Introduction | 1 |
| Chapter 1 - The History in Our Cells | 5 |
|     Family environment and birth imprints | 7 |
|     Injuries that are easy to ignore | 9 |
|     Pandora's Box of Suppressed Emotions | 13 |
|     Reflections of Personality and Psyche | 15 |
| Chapter 2 - Patterns of Expectation | 21 |
|     Self-image | 25 |
|     Modifying unrealistic expectations | 28 |
|     Confronting medical murkiness | 35 |
| Chapter 3 - Making Decisions Conscious | 39 |
|     Subconscious factors in decision-making: | 40 |
|         The unknown, Time & money, Stress, Fear, Negative self-talk, Pressure | |
|     Discerning types of pain: | 58 |
|         Ischemia, Numbness, Irritated trigger points | |
|         Headaches - tension, vascular, migraines; nausea | |
|         Dull aches, sharp, stinging pain, emotional | |
| Chapter 4. - Establishing a Baseline | 67 |
|     Getting a sense of things while sitting | 68 |
|     Negotiating torsion | 71 |
|     Sitting as a global event | 75 |
|     The eyes have it | 77 |

| | |
|---|---|
| Chapter 5 - Somatic In-sights | 80 |
| Entering the Deep Body | 83 |
| Biophotons | 85 |
| Increasing coherence | 87 |
| The eye of a storm in an injury | 92 |
| Being your own detective | 94 |
| Connecting the dots | 97 |
| Pairing for electrical, energetic, and fluid flow | 102 |
| Finding your baseline and balance while standing | 106 |
| Organizing the core | 110 |
| Pairing key locations as context for the brain | 114 |
| Creating cellular space | 118 |
| Opening space in the core | 120 |
| Healing the last percentages | 128 |
| About the Author | 134 |

# Acknowledgements

I'd like to express eternal gratitude for the multitude of teachers
and somatic pioneers whose practices and transmissions have
transformed the future possibilities in the arts, in the spirit,
and in our health and well-being for generations to come.
And a special thanks to Dr. Tom Hanna, who showed
up at the perfect time to start this somatic exploration
process that has taken on a life of its own
as it continues to transform mine.

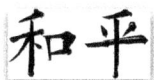

I'd also like to express sincere appreciation for all of the talented
International photographers on Pexels and Pixabay who were kind
enough to offer their wonderful images that are shown here in this
text for use to the public. Your generosity made the creation of
this body of work so much more fun and colorful, adding the
visual vocabulary to enhance the words.

# Preface

Suresha Hill has been known to me both in a personal and professional capacity for 25 years. I have always been struck by her kindness of being and sweetness of heart. Her life path has delved deeply into the spiritual, moving, and healing arts. This latest book is a personal account of a somatic journey which is unparalleled. Suresha takes us with her on a deep inquiry as to what self-healing is and how it takes place. Through her life experience and study of eastern and western spiritual healing arts she has opened up a path of self-discovery. This book shows us the how of 'being awareness', inside ourselves on a somatic bodily level is the key for health, healing and well-being. Suresha invites us to reclaim our somatic sovereignty through a very personal account of how she achieved just that, and used every injury as an opportunity for self-healing, self-organization, and growth. A must read for practitioner, student, and anyone who is interested in transformation.

Brian Siddhartha Ingle N.D., D.O., Osteopath

Osteopath, Naturopath, Hanna Somatic Educator, Feldenkrais Teacher.
The Ingle Institute for Somatic Education (IISE)

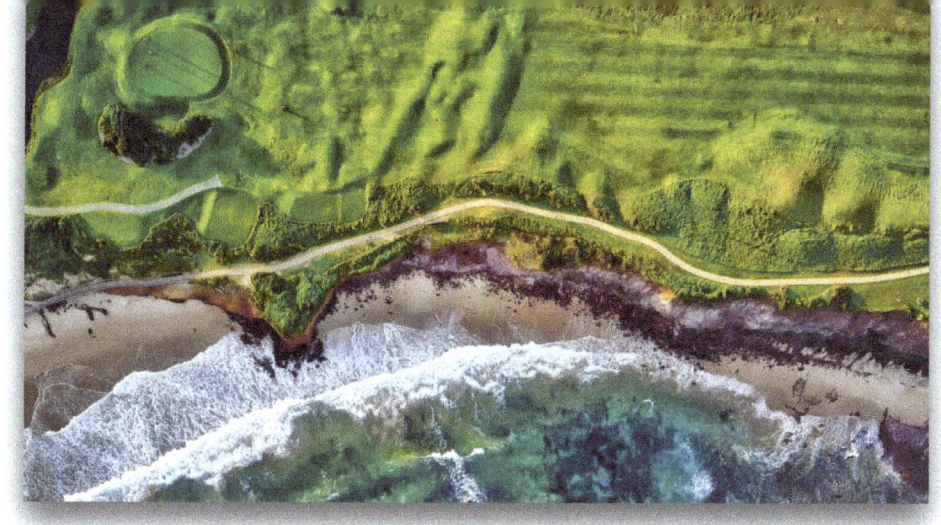

# Introduction

As I sit here today, I can hardly believe how much stress and trauma I've experienced in my lifetime. What's even more amazing is that I've healed from them all. From falls, car accidents, athletic injuries, various types of abuse, and concussions, to surgeries, race, gender, and creed injustices, hardly any type of wounding pain was left out. This volume focuses on the many lessons learned from the series of more than 50 layers of scarring experienced and resolved. Some were minor, some major, and everything in between. The challenge was in finding a way to heal, rather than to just feel better. Feeling better usually means to go on with your life as soon as it stops hurting. There are many ways that emotional, psychological, and physical injuries stop hurting as the body learns to adapt and continue functioning pretty well on the surface before an event has fully healed.

For the most part we prefer to move forward even when we know something isn't fully healed. It took quite a while for me to realize that there were many changes happening with each type of injury beneath the surface. They affected the way the body communicated with itself and contributed to several other mishaps that were then more complicated to heal. The learning process revealed the fact that injuries can be cumulative and interconnected. The way that they stack upon one another may not be obvious when you continue in a robust physical and athletic life. It can appear like there's an endless resiliency because the body may be masking the cumulative strain.

It might be hiding in elevated blood pressure, headaches, auto-immune issues, fibromyalgia, cancer, heart disease, addictions, eating disorders, and a host of other symptoms that have been displaced from their origin. that's the assumption when we're young. Dr. Van der Kolk, in "The Body Keeps the Score" focuses on the neurobiological changes that trauma produces that lead to PTSD. There are, however, millions of other cases where unresolved trauma has been shown to cause many other conditions, several of which are debilitating. For healthy folks who are super active, physical wounds seem to heal almost before you can tell anyone about it; in days or a few weeks tops. The body adapts to the scar tissue from a physical injury and we keep going as if nothing happened; it's hardly noticeable. Emotional wounds are another story, as is chronic stress. The mind suppresses emotional injuries and we keep going, not fully aware that every future experience is altered by those repressed wounds; not knowing that they inhibit the complete healing of our physical injuries or surgeries.

Consequences of choosing to 'feel better' or move forward aren't on your mind because you aren't aware of the adaptations. You may not feel them because they're subconscious, and because the young live more in the moment and those moments often don't seem connected. In fact, the part of the brain that connects them isn't fully developed yet. As we get older, we really can't help but notice the reduced adaptability, but chalk it up to aging. At some undisclosed point in time, that 'last straw' injury happens and adaptations have maxed out. Countless patients exclaim, "But I was only tying my shoe!" when excruciating back pain reveals that a disc 'suddenly' herniated, or a frozen shoulder seems to come out of nowhere.

You wouldn't realize that a current disc injury was related to several types of stress and strain that happened when you were young. You may not connect that the current insomnia, anxiety or depression started decades earlier either. One patient who'd gotten a frozen shoulder after a slight bump into a door only saw progress when she realized it was related to an emotional trauma in her family. That's why I'm writing this book; because I've seen so many cases where a recent condition doesn't resolve until the earlier connection is made. It was also true for me. What stood out initially was that the more recent injuries took longer than usual to heal. I made a mental note, but kept going at a breakneck pace. I wasn't ignoring my body or the signs that things were changing - quite the opposite. I was continually involved in self-care, and was feeling better and better, but there were still some missing pieces.

I didn't want that sluggish response in my system to be the new normal, and didn't want to blame it on aging. This curiosity into why things in my body were changing led to many explorations and discoveries that took time to unravel. I made many mistakes along the way even though I'd spent years studying the body, the psyche, energetic systems, and anything I could think of, as you could tell from the earlier volumes. Still, there were some sticky places inside that led to an elongated healing process that could have been avoided. This volume is straight talk on how to benefit from my mistakes as well as providing some insights along the way.

It's understandable that if you haven't studied the body and how it functions that the idea of taking charge of your own well-being and recovery process seems daunting. That's why I want to walk through it step-by-step covering all the bumps in the road that made my recovery process more difficult than it needed to be. I'll also get into what would have never been uncovered without the hours and hours of contemplation in those long nights without sleep, and working with thousands of clients over a few decades. Maybe you'll notice similar patterns in your own body, and be spared living in chronic discomfort that you've accepted as the new norm.

After years of feeling better, I only realized in October of 2019 that there was more healing to do. My body hadn't yet forgotten about the list of earlier incidents; it was still compensating and was functioning on a risky edge that was much more fragile that I thought. After a light to moderate workout at the gym, I was doing a little cool down stretching, leaning backwards over a large exercise ball when it took off and rolled me into the wall head first. I'd already had several blows to the head, so my first thought was, "Are you kidding me?" By then it seemed like there was some deeper reason that I'd continued to have head injuries; it just felt so surreal by that time. This incident helped me to see that the previous recovery efforts were still vulnerable to relapse. The pain that ensued in the following months exacerbated nearly every injury pattern I'd ever had. That was a shocker!

Now I'm really asking, "What is the key to complete healing, whereby the injury history has been resolved in every layer of my system that it's been stored in? What is keeping this memory matrix in place?" Toward the end of volume 6 there were so many 'aha's' and discoveries of new places to look, I really thought the quest was over. I felt 90% clear of every sort of trauma that had taken place and was excited to see where that last 10% was hiding. This last incident took me back down to 70%. It made it clear that there was still some thread that tied all the incidents of the history together, that when pulled, could still trigger them like a strand of Christmas lights that got plugged in. Was that strand a nerve fiber? A region of the brain? Connective tissue? I became determined to find out.

I'd never seen my neck go into the spiraling patterns it became compelled to do after this impact. The pile-on effect was creating new distortions that were boggling to unwind. If the body's memory of prior injuries was still this fresh and easy to reinstall, I had more to learn about the reeducation process, as well as how to reorganize and minimize the past imprints. Emotional scars from the past had been rewritten as far as my brain and heart were concerned, or so I thought. What about the cells, the fascia? Were there other areas of memory that I'd missed?

I once overheard a chiropractor I worked for say to a patient, "Don't settle for less than 100%". That last pain cycle reinvigorated the courage to find a way past the scary type of pain the October injury triggered, and into a quest for that 100%. It felt like every cell and the intelligence of the Universe was participating with me in this quest. It worked. I hope you feel the same way after reading this account of the harrowing journey from a recalculated 70% healed in October, to 98% healed by May 2020. By the end of writing this volume I hope to be able to say that all injuries are so reorganized away from injury patterns that they cannot be re-triggered. Possibly the other most rewarding aspect of this process besides healing, is the fact that the Intelligence that lives through us and through the body, increases in awareness simultaneously. I trust that if you're the type to buy this book, the journey will be as fascinating and rewarding for you as it has been for me.

**Merriam-Webster Dictionary**

**Fulcrum** - **a**. *a prop; the support about which a lever turns;*
**b**. *one that supplies capability for action*

*"Fulcrums are spatially related to the midline. Fulcrums are doorways between worlds."*

Dr. James Jealous, *An Osteopathic Odyssey*, 2015

*"Therapeutic processes that work through the body in present time, mediated by the prefrontal cortex, give access to real healing. Simply paying attention to sensation in the body can have this affect."*

Franklyn Sills, "Craniosacral Biodynamics - Volume 2; The Primal Midline and the Organization of the Body"

# Chapter 1

## The History in Our Cells

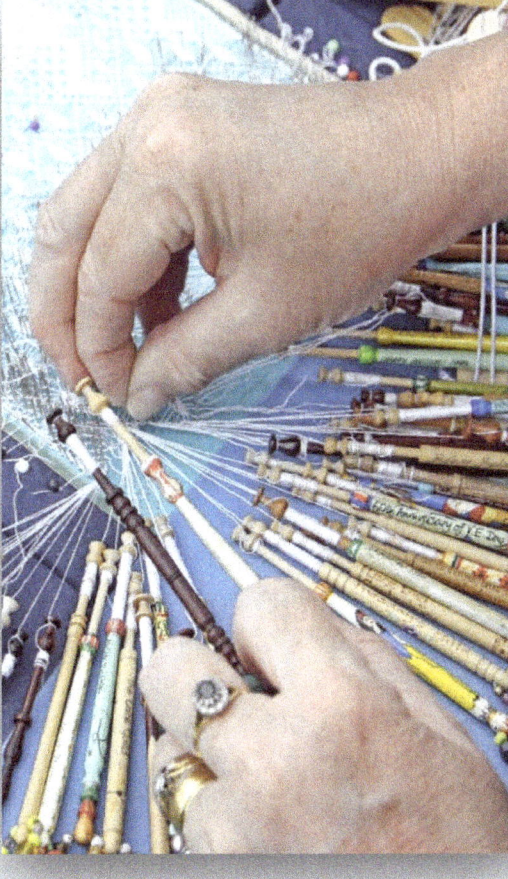

Our experiences weave a colorful, rich tapestry into the underlying framework of how and who we are genetically and culturally predisposed to be. Our bodies do an amazing job of pulling from threads of fundamental movement patterns so we can effectively walk, run, skip, write, draw, eat, ride bikes, climb trees, ski, wash dishes, and so many daily activities that we've become accustomed to. Every experience is being processed on some level whether conscious or unconscious. Experiences have a form that the body is using to process them, and likely have a 'tag' that the body uses to categorize, process, distribute, and store them.

Emotions have been tagged by Candace Pert (Molecules of Emotion, 1997) as ligands, or a type of protein that has form and function. They can then attach to certain receptor sites that may trigger neurotransmitters and act as a form of information for the system. Thoughts are believed to be transmitted across nerve cells with an electrical charge, (McCrae,"*Neuroscientists Have Followed a Thought as it Moves Through the Brain*"; *Science Alert*, January 2018) which are also able to stimulate the production of neurotransmitters and presumably, stress hormones.

Our genes store many hereditary physical, mental, and health traits or predispositions that may express under certain conditions. Children often take on posture and gait patterns, personality and behavior tendencies, and more from their parents and grandparents. Imagine how small these bytes of information need to be in order to be stored in our cells, coded and filed, waiting to be called into action according to its role in the situation at hand. The main thing to remember, is that thoughts and emotions are also processed by our bodies and make a big difference in health outcomes. How we respond to every experience is key to well-being because our bodies are not only listening, but are also being guided by us.

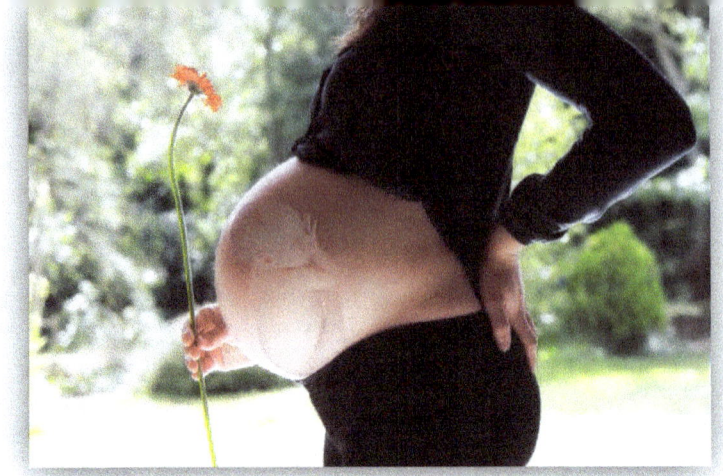

These complex systems are continually responsive to life's experiences, as well as being shaped by them and by other factors we are still discovering. In my way of thinking as well as those in the field of neuroscience, the brain is as much, if not more of a reflection and coordinator of what we experience, as it is a director of how our experiences unfold. Even its directions are learned. The extent to which the brain functions in one capacity over another may very well be the extent to which we step in as the mediator between objective or outer, and inner, subjective realities. You are ideally in between the two.

We are mammals by design and bound in some ways to that evolutionary puzzle. However, even instinctual, sensory, and tactile information passes by the prefrontal cortex before executing the final action. Every parent, older sibling, and babysitter knows that children have to be trained to make safe and socially appropriate decisions. It doesn't come naturally. We know that early wiring is also dictated by environment. The numbers of neurons that link to the prefrontal cortex versus the hind brain for fight/flight activation is determined by how much stress the mother is experiencing during pregnancy and lactation periods. There is latitude everywhere you look in terms of our human tendencies and capacities.

It's not that we're completely tabula rasa - a blank slate - as our cells are assigned a certain blueprint which they follow for the basic rules of form and function. Our stomach knows exactly how to break down food, our lungs know how to breathe. We are, however, gifted with a biological marvel that is so open to learning that it can even overcome autonomic functions. Some yogis have learned to alter their breath, heartbeat, temperature, and excretions. Reflexive survival tendencies like fear and anger, responses which are also learned or pre-programmed, can be overridden. We are not altogether a 'ghost in the machine' even if early life has created a hyper-vigilant, survival orientation. There is still the potential to rewrite the narrative or switch neurological tracks so that our responses travel down a preferred pathway. As long as we can expand in awareness, change is possible. We are increasing in awareness of ourselves as the fulcrum, at the same time the body develops more awareness of itself.

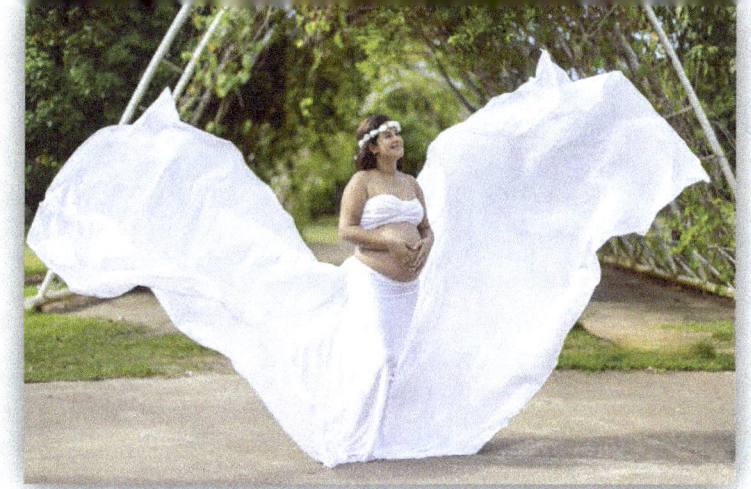

It's the closest answer I have to the age-old question of whether the sound of a tree falling happens if no one is there listening to it. Your body will be making sounds in response to your experiences whether or not you are present. But if you're not present, a change won't be either. Your system will draw from genetic predispositions and learned habits in an automatic, unconscious way. If you are present, many new options are available for how it will respond. Developing presence and discernment in awareness takes practice, because a lot of our attention placement is also learned or predisposed. It's pretty much making the effort to wake up out of a trance.

All it really takes to change neurological tracks is desire, motivation, and intention. There are a few things that can keep the train from leaving the station of habit, that also make it hard to pierce the reasons why it's not leaving. Let's cover some of the reasons that could be blocking new behavior even when the desire is there. Most of these initial reasons include experiences that are inherently subcortical and prior to the development of the 'observer' who is able to witness and question the lack of movement in a new direction. If you can't see clearly, something in you will keep you from changing; something you can't put your finger on.

## Family history and birth imprints

Genetics is definitely a factor in how we form as an embryo and fetus. It leaves basic imprints that are unalterable, such as height, skin, hair and eye color, and shape of the musculoskeletal system. There is much evidence to show that the environment of the womb is carried into the fetus in forms like drugs, smoking, diet, illnesses, or stress status of the mother and family. These impressions and influences will be difficult to identify initially. Some may have been fortunate enough to have a mother who strolled beaches in the wind with flowers in her hair during their pregnancy, but most didn't. If you're in a younger generation, you're in luck. More children have had mothers who meditated and took yoga classes to help their body and mind to be a gracious, calm host for the incoming soul, and they also report easier times with labor and delivery.

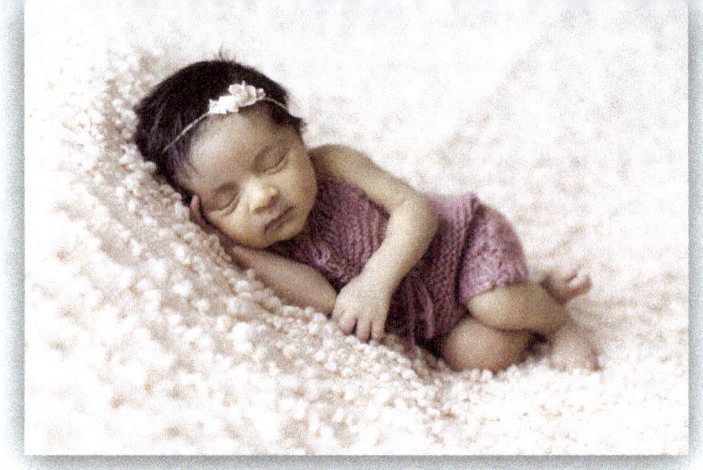

Recently mothers have been electing to have home births, water births, and natural births without anesthesia or drugs. They're surrounded by loved ones in a calm, quiet space with music, soft lighting, and midwives. Studies of water births consistently report fewer complications, less pain and pain medication or epidurals, and shorter labors. This constitutes 1% of all births. At least 40% are C-sections, or are induced. Mao and Jing discovered in 2005 after two decades of observation, that infants born using C-section were more likely to resist intimate touching with their mothers, had reduced sensory perception, reduced visual spatial relationships capacity, and reduced visual memory.

An extensive Australian study of 500,000 women and their children over a period of 13 years demonstrated that C-section babies had the highest rates of metabolic disorders by the time they were five years-old, as well as higher rates of respiratory infections, of metabolic disorders and dermatitis among babies born with *any* type of birth intervention. There were no mothers with risk factors for having the C-section in the study. Genes that respond to the stress of labor and delivery by boosting immune function are not switched on in a C-section. In addition, the beneficial bacteria from the vaginal delivery that is protective for the child's health is also missing, making the child more vulnerable to allergies, diabetes, infections, and obesity. (The Conversation, *"How birth interventions affect babies' health in the short and long term";* March, 2018)

Along with physiological factors that can imprint in the early stages of being human, personality disorders can develop later in life when the mother was exposed to high stress levels during her pregnancy. This Finnish study done by the British Journal of Psychiatry followed the children of 3600 women into adulthood, and reported that these adults were almost 10 times more likely to experience depression, alcohol or substance abuse, anxiety, emotional instability, or antisocial behavior. (Health, *"Stress in pregnancy makes child personality disorder more likely"* September 2019). Studies have also shown that children born by vaginal delivery have higher cognitive skills (Scientific Reports, Sept. 2017). In addition, infant vaccines have been linked to high blood pressure, connective tissue

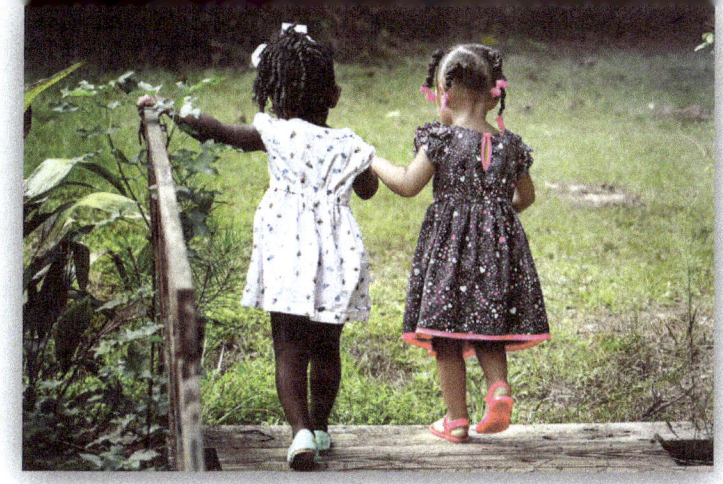

disease, liver damage, fever, chills, autism, lupus, vomiting, dermatitis and more. There is also a percentage of women for whom the pregnancy, labor and delivery processes are so overwhelming that they develop PTSD, anxiety, or depression., whereby they are not available to bond with their new infant.

Experiences that are subconscious from the preverbal time in your life and therefore fairly ingrained, can feel like something you're 'born with' and stuck with. They could be affecting why the train for healing isn't leaving the station. On the way to the fullness of healing, it's possible to bump up against these early, sticky bits when the more salient and more recent injuries begin to discharge. Your body will have a language to let you know that the sticky bits are there, but also asking your parents about those years could be very helpful in unraveling the mystery.

## Injuries that are easy to ignore

If I had a nickel for every time a client said, "But that was a long time ago!" I'd have had an island vacation by now. I've rarely if ever met someone who believes or realizes that something from infancy, toddler years, elementary school years, and particularly birth trauma is still affecting their well-being unless they've specifically studied the subject. I remember a few instances during Primal Scream Therapy (yes, I did that one), and in the Rebirthing Training (this one was total bliss!) when the sounds I was making and the shapes my body went into were absolutely bizarre. They were reminiscent of infancy and the deep squeeze of the birth canal as my body was being pushed out. It was so primordial that there weren't words to accompany the sounds and movements. The cognitive brain wasn't developed yet, but reliving it as a discharge of old cellular trauma was enlivening and relieving. It made a believer out of me.

It's easy to ignore birth trauma because you have no memory of it, but there is a sense when something feels off. If you have that feeling, asking your mother about the circumstances surrounding her pregnancy and your birth could confirm it. I'm not sure those impressions would have surfaced without those processes, but also

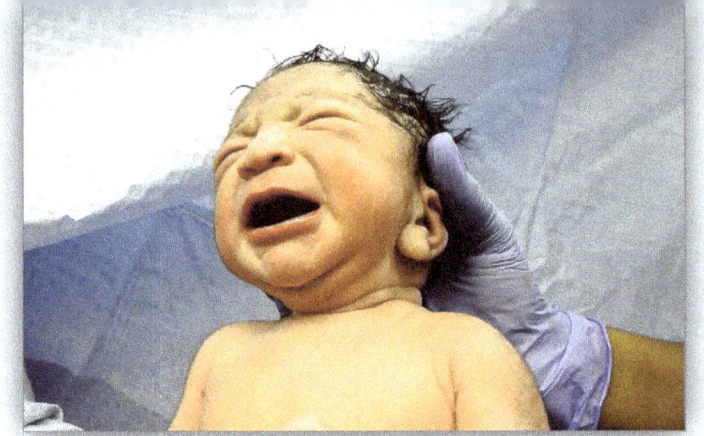

trust that the body's intelligence finds a way. Just follow that inkling and seek a gentle form of treatment. Don't worry about going back into the intensity of it. There's a difference between releasing and reliving an experience. Remember, it's not a tiny, 6 pound infant's body experiencing it, but a capable adult intentionally going into the therapeutic process who can modulate responses in the context of the release; not in a context of re-experiencing trauma. Cranial sacral therapy can unhinge some of these deeper memories, and Ray Castellino offers programs to release birth imprinting. Although the memories are remote, people who need this type of healing often know it on some level.

If you knew for sure that those hidden wounds were shaping your brain, your personality, your health, and every relationship you have, you might jump the hurdle. You'd make it a point to acquire the skills to navigate and nurture the complexity of our own body, mind, and heart. We need those strong, numbing experiences to be discharged as soon as possible! The release of those early traumas opens the numbness and yields entry into the subtle, balancing, healing characteristics of Spirit. It rewires your nervous system and changes your perception of how you are as a human.

Young people aren't in touch enough with their bodies, nor do they have the language or experience to know that they need more help. They may even say, "I'm fine." It doesn't mean it's true. Just like when adults use that phrase to really say, "I don't want to think about it right now." You as an adult can decide against making choices that are numbing or that sweep things under the rug, for you and for your children. It's easy to avoid or ignore embarrassing hurts and traumas; in fact, we usually prefer to avoid them. Ignoring your health is a recipe for disaster. It's like dismantling your house one brick at a time, then feeling horrified that it collapsed. The only reason we do that is because no one lets us know how it works. I had no idea what was coming. It's been shown that emotional traumas in young life can become inflammatory conditions, personality disorders, recurring

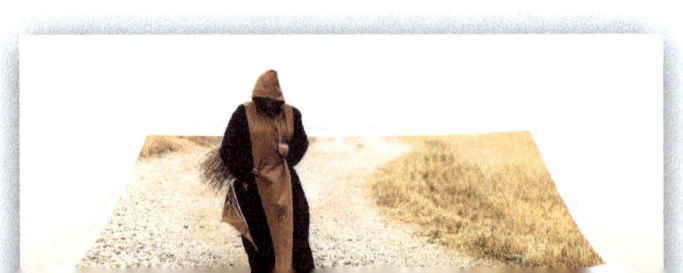

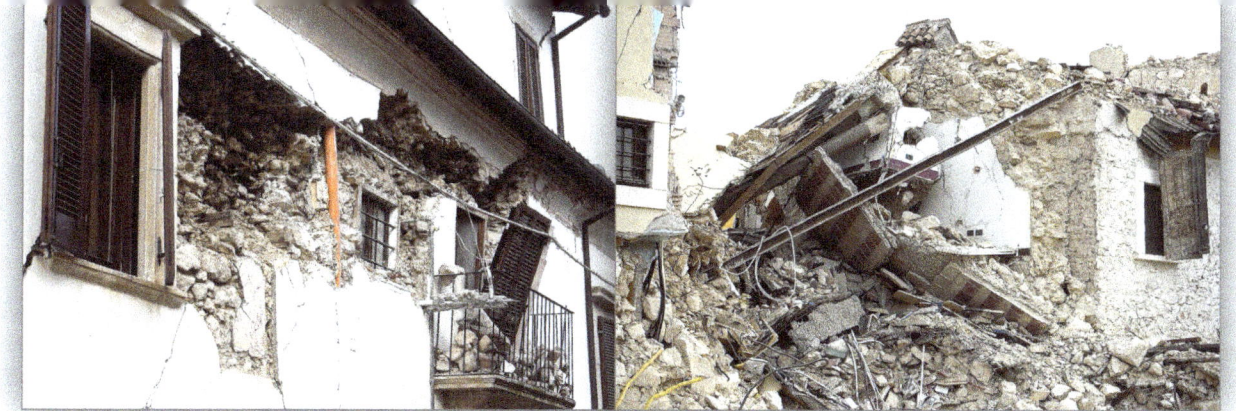

headaches, or self-harming issues. Harvard Health Publishing printed an article in 2019 that listed heart attack, stroke, cancer, PTSD, depression, psychiatric disorders, obesity, and other health issues as being related to childhood trauma. This is no small load to carry. Every waking and sleeping moment is being formed by those traumas that act as information shaping your system's response to anything and everything.

I don't remember the umbilical hernia surgery at three years old, but it turned out to be a key restriction that made a huge impact on digestion, and on tension patterns out into my hips. It may have contributed to the sciatica that developed in my twenties, and the weakness that contributed to the disc injury. There is still a numb sensation in the area of my forehead with those swing set stitches, and when subsequent head injuries were up for healing, that area of my head became sore again; a real focal point for constriction. The surgeries I had at 3, 5, and 9 years-old were minor, yet left scar tissue that revealed itself to be a significant factor later in life. I only realized years later that overcoming symptoms of whiplash and concussions were being influenced by those earlier surgeries.

The laparoscopic surgery at 28 years of age was influential as well. It tied into the earlier hernia scar. The tonsillectomy created extra tension in the deep fascia in my throat that a later whiplash triggered. The little procedure inside my nasal cavity at 5 years-old laid down extra bone that created irritation whenever I wore sunglasses or reading glasses after a later concussion jarred the injury back to the surface. In this sense, injuries of all kinds can become timeless. I also realized much later that scars interfere with and alter communication from the body to the brain.

As folks roll into their teens and twenties, mishaps are much easier to recall, but somehow we have that, "I am Invincible!" thing going on so it doesn't register that hitting the water hard while surfing, or the snowpack while snowboarding, or diving into home plate to win the baseball game could impact present day discomforts. For one thing, there's so much adrenaline moving through your system that the incident barely registers as being painful. For another thing, you're in the midst of an ongoing activity that's fast paced and demands total focus. You're being caught up in the energy of the moment, then the next, and the next moment.

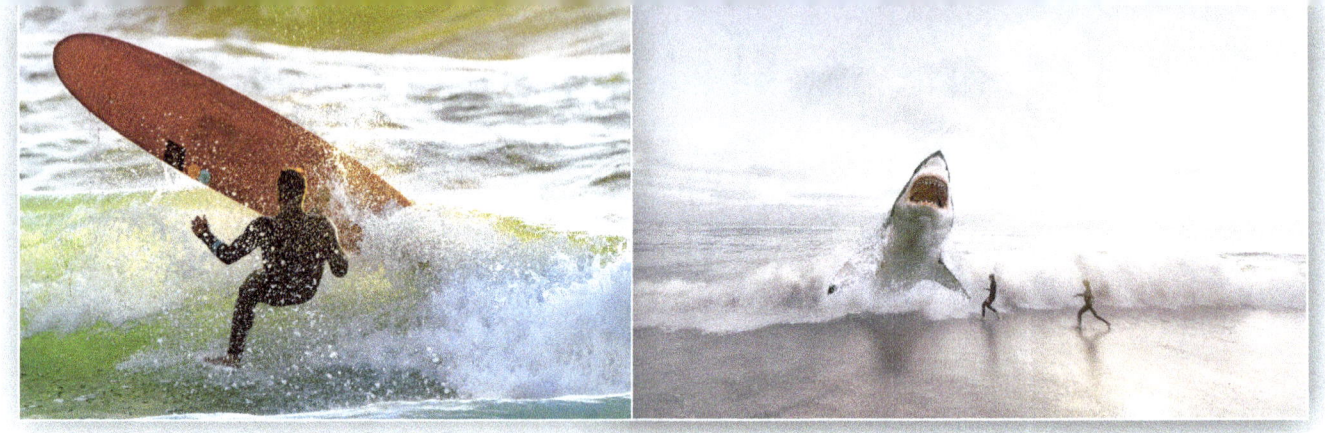

While being in a contact sport in the form of karate for 13 years, we'd spent a lot of time training to hit and get hit, so we were in pretty good shape. We expected to be sore the next day, because we continually pushed our limits. If there was a wound, it felt better so quickly that it wasn't given a second thought. They all seemed to disappear into the energy of the next exercise or fight. These types of injuries and repetitive impacts are easy to ignore because for all we could tell, everything was still normal. If there was a little stiff place here or there, you're trained to 'work through it' and keep going. It was 'normal' to be a little sore most of the time.

Slowing down physical activity later in life definitely makes those little stiff places stand out, and we call it 'getting older'. With that change of focus in activity, the energy circulates in a different way in the system; things slow down. Then the places that used to retain fluidity begin to catch and stiffen and are noticeable. These are the sharks of the deep that come back to bite you later in life. Whether it's football, soccer, horseback riding, falls from motorcycles or bikes, car accidents, skiing mishaps, falls on ice, or whatever the source of injury, Hundreds of clients come in when an old injury flares up, but leave it be as soon as it stops hurting; as soon as it feels better.

I'm encouraging you to take a deep dive into your system so you can seek out and work out the stiff, adhesive places and treat each one as though it's a nail in your proverbial coffin. Most doctors will not try to heal you, or encourage you to heal. They will try to help you feel better enough to function. You have to be your own ally here. Even if you'd had a hard time knowing what it's like to love yourself, love the freedom of being able to continue to do all the things you love to do. If you don't make the effort to heal all the way, some, if not all of those activities will be out of your life. Luckily, at some point I stopped the fighting aspect of the external art, and headed into the internal martial arts like chi kung.

Hopefully after reading this, you won't wait until your system runs out of bandwidth and starts expressing major symptoms. Hopefully, you will seek treatments that return you to 100% as soon as you notice or remember the trauma or injury. You can't imagine what an incredible return you would receive on this investment, but I hope you'll take the leap and find out.

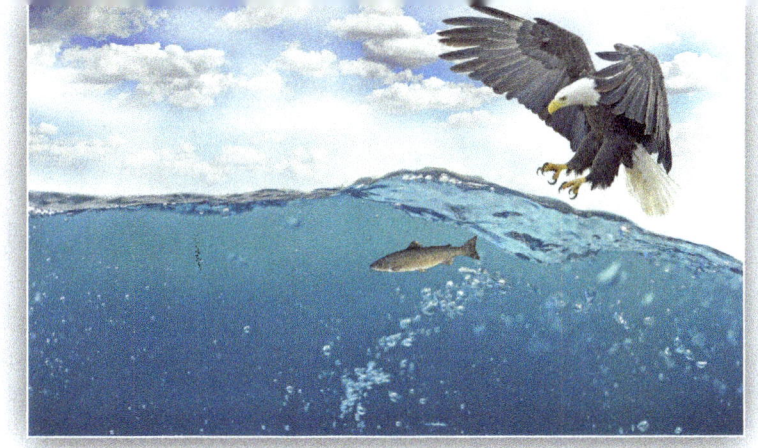

## Pandora's box of suppressed emotion

One of the easiest categories of experiences to forget is the box of stuff we wished had never happened. There are also those ongoing daily life stressors that we do remember, but wish we could forget. They're a little different from events that leave scars. Birth trauma, surgeries, falls, and accidents are singular incidents that can easily be ignored because they seem to be in the past. Daily life stressors are another source of emotional injury that can easily become somaticized - held in your body - or wind up as part of a personality disorder. The brain hasn't fully matured until mid-twenties, and even then, a stable processing system for powerful emotions may not be fully developed. Many studies have shown that early emotional injury is related to health issues later in life. A.C.E. is the acronym for Adverse Childhood Events, which, during a Kaiser study of over 17,000 adults in the 1990's, was shown to be predictive in our health and well-being by middle age.

The adverse events include such things as abuse, neglect, divorce or separation of parents, alcoholism, or a major illness of a parent. It was shown that childhood trauma was a root cause of major illness and could potentially shorten a lifespan by as much as 20 years and increase *risk of death by all diseases.* A 2008 study published in the Malaysian Journal of Medical Sciences showed that chronic stress suppresses the immune system, raises the risk of infection, diabetes, asthma, ulcerative colitis, arteriosclerosis, psychiatric illness, and the development of cancer. This study cites that the European Agency for Safety and Health attribute 50% of absenteeism at work being stress-related, and 80-90% of industrial accidents being due to inability to cope with stress. In 2017 U.S and European physicians find 75-90% of doctor visits attributable to stress-related symptoms.

It's very rare that a child will be able to admit to abuse or know that they should. Women are just now speaking out about abuses that happened many years earlier. Men are more reluctant to speak up or to seek treatment, and if the abuses are early enough, it could take decades before they are exposed or admitted. It took at least twenty years to tell my mother what happened with our babysitters, and

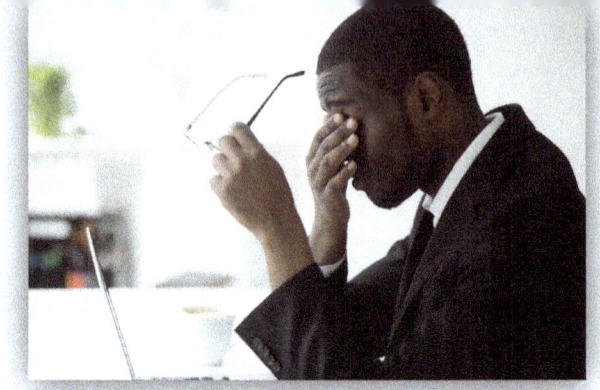

twenty years after the fact, my daughter shared how cruel her babysitter was. I was shocked because she seemed like the nicest person you'd ever want to meet. Consider that trauma is in the eye of the beholder, and a harsh punishment, neglect, or even witnessing harsh treatment of others can seem traumatic for a vulnerable child when no one is there to guide them through it.

Divorce is usually preceded by a long period of discomfort in the household, affecting children and adults alike. It might not be difficult to explain the 'why' to children, but on another level, the separation of their parents remains difficult to accept. Here's another place where guidance through processing the situation, both in your own system as well as for the rest of the family is key. You remaining neutral as much as possible, as the fulcrum around which the entire experience will revolve, determines how the unavoidable event will play out in your system and in the lives of those who shared the loss. You being able to remain in neutral acceptance of what you know to be the best decision, even though it won't feel good or feel fair, is the best way for your body and mind not to harbor the stress.

Chronic stress has been shown to limit the body's ability to exert hormonal control over its inflammatory response creating more susceptibility to disease, and causing diseases like auto-immune disease, asthma, and cardiovascular disease. (Carnegie Mellon Institute, Science Daily, "*How Stress Influences Disease - Study Reveals Inflammation as the Culprit*", April 2012) The study also revealed that the symptoms of a common cold were a side-effect of the body's response of the immune system fighting inflammation, but not the cause of the symptoms as we are currently discovering with what we've called a 'virus'.

Is it no wonder then, that tens of millions of people are on medication for pain, anxiety, insomnia and depression, along with tens of millions who are self-medicating with alcohol and other substances? These stresses, tensions, and imbalances in biochemistry are all sitting in the cells, and likely have been for quite some time. These tensions are part of what can create restrictions and distortions of what would otherwise be a natural flow of fluids, fascia, joint articulations, organ and gland function, just like early injuries can. Weight gain and slowed wound healing have also been associated with stress. I'll never forget the woman who told me she gained 100 pounds after her husband and daughter died in a car accident.

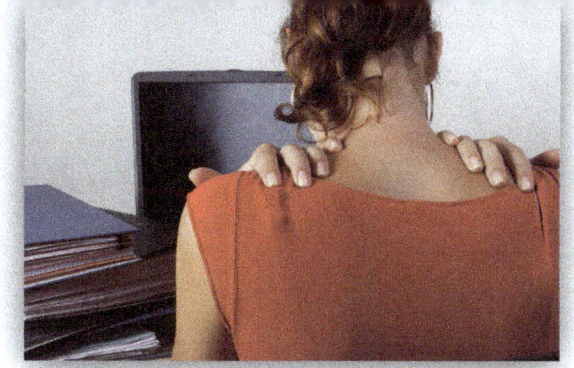

Some things are hard to accept, hard to process, and will require patient, gentle self-inquiry in all those tender places inside where the trauma lives. Luckily, there are forms of somatic bodywork, body-based therapies, hypnotherapy and breath therapy, as well as active meditations that can greatly help suppressed or numbed emotions to be released from your system. Quite a few of the somatic pioneers had chronic conditions both mentally and physically that kept them from fully participating in their lives, some more serious than others.

Elsa Gindler had tuberculosis, F. Matthias Alexander had chronic laryngitis as an actor, and Gerda Alexander suffered from endocarditis - inflammation of the inner membrane of the heart. Each was able to see a remarkable improvement in their mental, emotional, and physical status by mindfully exploring how they were using their bodies in daily life. Andrew Still, the father of osteopathy, was able to save lives during a black diphtheria outbreak using manual therapy alone. Milton Trager reported instances where cancer was cured in his clients through using joint mobilization combined with a 'hook' up to the Higher Power by the practitioner.

Mental and emotional well-being, and physical health can be addressed internally, regardless of the source of trauma. All experiences find a way to be processed by the cells, but realizing that *memories have a tangible form* provides the impetus to find a healthy method for their release. As you learn your body's vocabulary, you will discover which form these memories have and where they live in you. Love can also make you feel better, and in some cases heal you. I had a client whose painful fibromyalgia symptoms were from the pain and grief cause by the death of her husband. It disappeared when she fell in love again. If it's not a simple, direct link like that, it likely will not erase all of the earlier imprints that reside in your body.

## Reflections of personality and psyche

Personality and psyche are fluid. Tendencies can develop from an early age based upon early experiences, but what can be learned has the potential to be unlearned. The home environment can have a tremendous impact on how a personality will express and how the psyche will be shaped. If there isn't a constant positive role model around, children will quite naturally imitate the figures in front of them, even if they're on the television or on video games. The American Academy of Child and

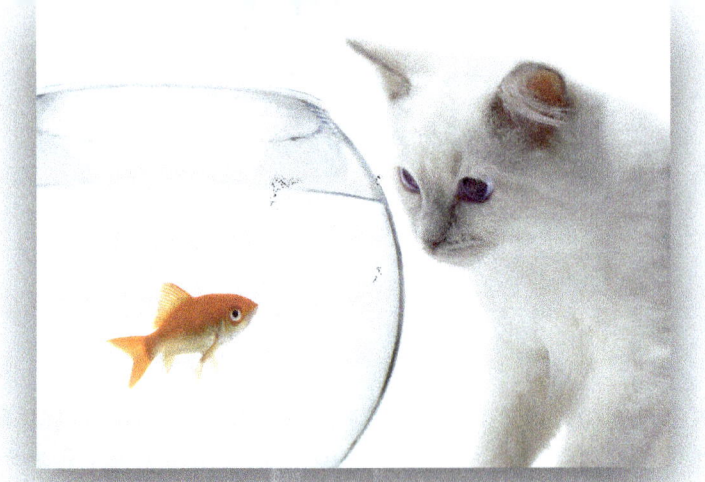

Adolescent Psychiatry stated in a 2015 report that, "Studies of children exposed to violent media have shown that they may become numb to violence, imitate the violence, and show more aggressive behavior. They go on to say, "Younger children and those with emotional, behavioral or learning problems may be more influenced by violent images." The same is true for adults, as the mean age of those playing video games is 30. Up to 90% of video games are violent. It's been a widely studied topic, with a few longitudinal studies of up to 5,000 participants find that playing regularly increases risky, aggressive behavior, and decreases desirable social behaviors like empathy. (Healthline, October 2018) Suffice to say that the brain and personality are regularly changing to reflect our activities.

When participating in extracurricular activities or sports, having compassionate handling around winning, losing, and good sportsmanship is also very valuable. Hormones do change according to the psyche's perception of success or failure, therefore how grades and academic performance are handled during our lives is a big part of self-perception and self-esteem. Even adult psyches can easily be reorganized according to the self-critical state that neurotransmitters take you to when the psyche feels defeated, unsuccessful, or like you let your teammates or family down. It's helpful to know that the brain's chemistry isn't the same as who you are, and that if you pat yourself on the back instead of giving in to the chemistry, you wouldn't have attached a negative self-concept to performance.

Children and adults are treated differently when they look or act dissimilar from their peers. Marginalized teens have a much higher drop-out rate, a higher rate of teen pregnancies, and are often on a fast track to juvenile court. Kids who are bullied at school or at home may begin to show signs of anxiety and depression, of learned helplessness and hopelessness. They often get worse grades, begin to act out or become withdrawn, and become ill more often - particularly with skin or intestinal problems. Eating and sleeping disorders may show up in youth under chronic stress, and in some cases, adolescents even commit suicide. Society has routinely used pharmaceuticals and talk therapy to treat behaviors, without solutions.

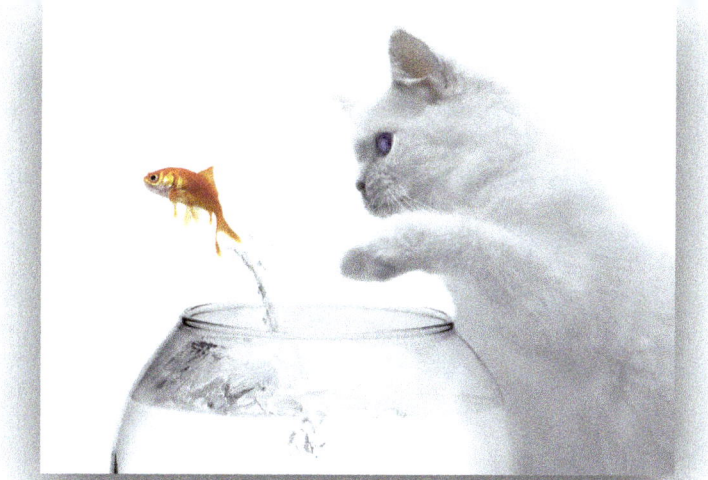

Victims of bullying as children including those who played both roles - being both the perpetrator and the victim - were much more likely to have the same psycho-emotional issues as adults and develop substance abuse problems. Unresolved childhood issues show up later in life on many fronts. The workplace has been established as a major source of stress for many people, likely being an easy trigger for early patterns to be repeated. A poll taken in 2017 by the American Osteopathic Association found that over 30% of the 2000 people polled had experienced bullying. The long-term effects included sleep loss, headaches, muscle pains, more frequent illnesses, eating disorders, high blood pressure, self-harming behavior, thyroid issues, and mood disorders.

What becomes of the bully? Although they don't seem to develop health issues as a result of their cruelty towards others, it's been shown that they can easily develop a personality disorder like that of a sociopath when in a position of power as an adult. Treatment by others and the perception of others as children can become internalized and stick to them as part of their identity. The good news is that any type of trauma is mediated by the orientation to it by the person receiving the rough treatment. The extent of the trauma is strongly influenced by the significant adults around at the time. For example, it's been shown that soldiers who had a superior officer in their unit who remained calm and led confidently with a steady hand were less likely to develop PTSD.

In the same way, when there was a supportive intervention for the bullied children, they were much less likely to suffer long-term consequences. A certain amount of stress and challenge strengthen us and teach us how to overcome hurdles and to handle the wide variety of situations that may come along. They also educate the immune system and the nervous system as to what they should be taking into consideration, and how best to adapt. Children and adults alike benefit from learning how to surf rough tides while staying in balance. It's very beneficial to learn how to manage one's own climate of emotional and mental turmoil as soon as you can. Then you won't wind up being your own bully or bullying others.

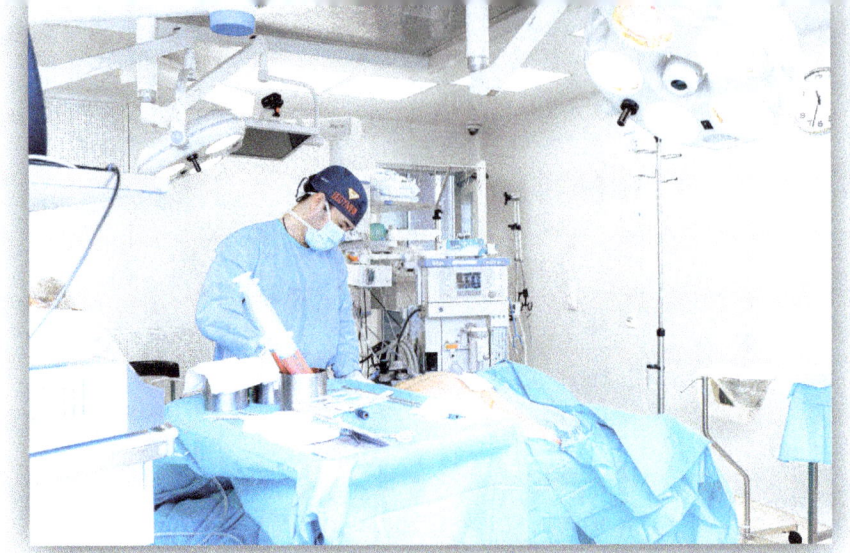

It's also key to realize that the mind, musculoskeletal system, neurophysiology, and heart are all related, and that you are their superior officer. You are the fulcrum around which experiences are perceived, organized, categorized, and stored. Just like for your muscles, if there isn't someone navigating an emotional experience mindfully, your brain will recruit familiar or predisposed patterns to use. The subconscious patterns often won't be the best, or even the most appropriate reaction to use, but it'll be out of your mouth before you can catch it. Physical reactions can be powerful in an emotional event, and when your brain sees the physical one, the psyche will produce cues from a fight/flight response like you're in danger unless you step in consciously to regulate the storm.

Your body will listen to the superior officer during an emergency unless an earlier trauma gets triggered. Even then, if you're mindful that something's been triggered and the situation in front of you isn't to blame, your system will still let go of an inappropriate reaction. Honestly, if someone had told me this when I was 30 years-old, I initially would have stared blankly because there was no foundation to build the new information upon. It would have sounded like a foreign language that I didn't have the vocabulary to. Repetition is key. That's one reason I'll be going over so many of the underlying tendencies that establish the basis for how the body languages within itself, and for how we can take part in the conversation; to help build that foundation.

There will be exceptions when neither the body nor the superior officer are on board, and that's the case during surgery. Anesthesia ties the hands of the body and shuts off its ability to respond. During a minor surgery I had a few decades ago, the surgeon mentioned afterwards that although I was knocked out with two forms of anesthesia, my body was still wriggling to avoid the knife. Probably still had a little martial arts defensive moves in the mix, even while unconscious. However, there is an impression of powerlessness that enters in when neither you nor your body can prevent the painful intrusion. It's a shock.

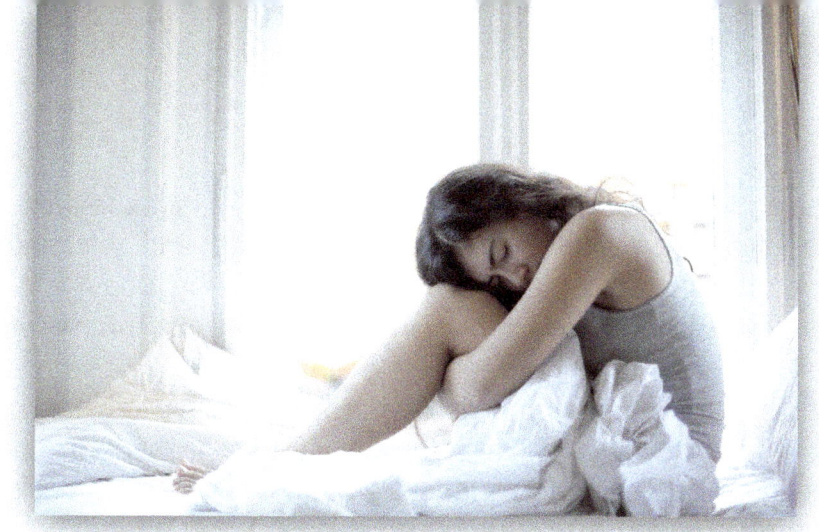

Although numbed, the impression stays in the cells in a certain way. Is it any surprise that the body can't get over it and come to resolution? The inflammatory status leads to arthritis at the site in so many cases when a joint is involved. In other areas of soft tissue, the information and energetic pathways are altered, as is the brain's perception of the area. There is a certain type of trauma associated with a surgical procedure that can take the area offline in a variety of ways, even after you feel better. Most of those limitations can be overcome with physical therapy. If it becomes a chronic issue, there's a chance the shock was not fully released and should be addressed with manual therapy.

Surgery is scary for many people, because it already has built in risks and you're unconscious and can't participate to boot. One of my relatives didn't survive a very minor hiatal hernia surgery due to a preventable allergic reaction to a medication. It's hard to forget that. You have to wonder if someone will miss that little detail in your chart that lists your allergies. Even if it goes fairly well and no foreign objects are left in your body, it is estimated that 33% of patients who spend more than 5 days in intensive care develop some, if not multiple forms of ICU psychosis. Some of the circumstances that induce the delirium can include isolation, pain, loss of control, constant medical interventions and monitoring, sensory overload by machines and noise, sleep deprivation, no windows in the room, and likely pre-existing stressors.

A long-time colleague of mine experienced this type of hysteria after a successful heart surgery. She was sedated to contain her hysteria, and was somewhat calmed by familiar music, but eventually her organs failed and she passed away. It always puzzled me that since these psychoses disappear when the patient leaves the ICU, why they kept her there for three weeks because she was hysterical. Unfortunately, she'd been on pain meds for years for earlier hip replacements that became arthritic. Then the pain meds for this surgery weren't working. These extra little insults to injury can also become unsettling for loved ones and become stored in memory fields as reasons to avoid medical attention.

Of course, many do survive surgery, but the entire hospital experience, along with whatever the initial injury was, need to be addressed and released before the healing can be complete. If there is preparation for the body and the psyche beforehand, I believe that many of the harmful impressions can be reduced, if not alleviated. Asking questions in advance of any procedure, like who might be the best surgeon and anesthesiologist for what you need done, what the surgeon's track record is, and how many times they've had to go back in soon after the original procedure is a good start. Bedside manner may be a consideration, but expertise and track record may be more important if you already have a support system in place.

Surgical nurses are often privy to details about who is known to have the best reputation for which procedure. It might be a good idea to also find out what the hospital's procedures are around their ICU; what the rooms look like, what to expect in the surgery's aftermath, what the visitation policies are, and so on, to minimize potentially shocking surprises. It could also be helpful to have plans for some type of somatic therapy session after your procedure to help the system decompress and reduce the likelihood of mini-traumas creating preventable issues. That said, the body has its timing and its wisdom. It may not be ready to release trauma and shock while it's still processing it. A reflexive 'freeze' may induce many types of contraction in different systems. Best to wait for a bit of thawing so flow is opened again and recovery methods will be best received.

It happens for some clients that they enter into many different types of treatments with a variety of practitioners for quite a while, until one day it seems like the magic happens. All rivers are pouring into the sea at the same moment and the elusive threads that have been holding a pattern in place expose themselves and let go. The weaver, the weave, the loom, and the unweaving become one in that moment. Even though there may be layers, it's an amazing feeling when you feel like you've uncovered and let go of an entire gestalt that was creating discomfort. There are times when the entire syndrome surfaces at the same time, but the more common scenario is when one piece comes up for air, then another, just like debris from a wreckage in an old plane crash that had sunk to the bottom of the sea.

There isn't an emotional component that has to be relived necessarily, but there is often fear that there will be. From the perspective of the shock of surgery, near the scar there could be a tad of anesthesia-like numbing, some trembling, jerking, and heat release with the discharge. The overwhelming sensation, however, is one of relief when the cells bring the shock to the surface, and allows the surrounding areas to awaken and regain participation with the rest of the body.

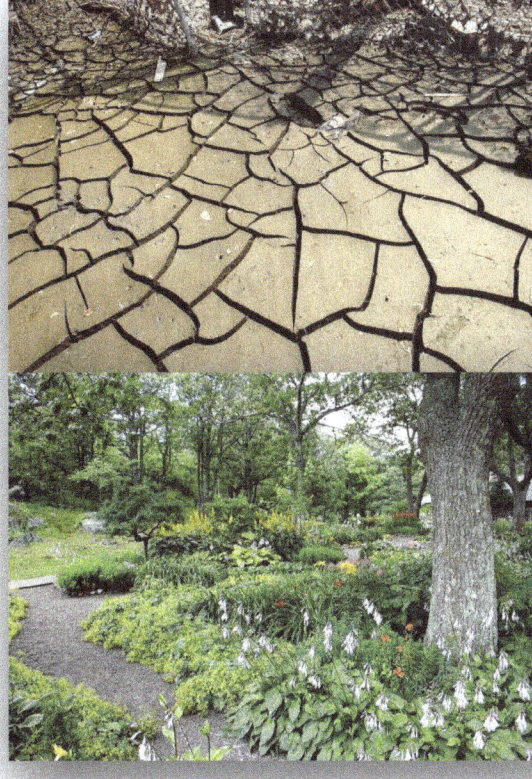

# Chapter 2

# Patterns of Expectation

Our personalities often contain patterns of belief and expectation that are so near and familiar, we hadn't taken a step back to enquire where they came from. Receiving praise and avoiding disapproval from those who matter to us are classic examples of how we bend to expectations outside of ourselves. Our own opinions tend to match the expectations of those we want the approval of. They can eventually become an internal voice that can be strict and harsh, or gently chiding but persistent, usually matching the person's voice we initially heard it from.

Young children are pretty wide open within their experiences, as ideas about life haven't taken hold yet, and the adults around us are still telling us how we're supposed to feel or not feel about things. It is pretty common to adopt the perspective of parents until the influence of peers act as a bridge to when our own opinions begin to form. Within whatever pattern that takes shape, nothing is set in stone. According to Bruce Lipton, cell biologist and author of "Biology of Belief" and "The Honeymoon Effect," our cells are often responding to what we subconsciously believe. They will change the shape of receptor sites to allow a messenger protein to bind in accordance with our expectations. Lipton flipped the script on the idea that we are heavily influenced by our genetics, and has most of modern science realizing that the expression of many genetic codes is heavily influenced by its environment, of which belief is a part. So it's not just thoughts and emotions, but beliefs also facilitate changes in our physiology, responding to you as the fulcrum.

The placebo effect is a perfect example of outcomes being linked to expectation. It's not a cut and dry causality however, as there are a few factors that have an impact on the degree to which the placebo is 'activated' in the mind of the person. One factor is the extent to which the source delivering the information is believable to the person, as in how confident they sound, how much of an authority they are in the mind of the person, and how many times or by how many other people there

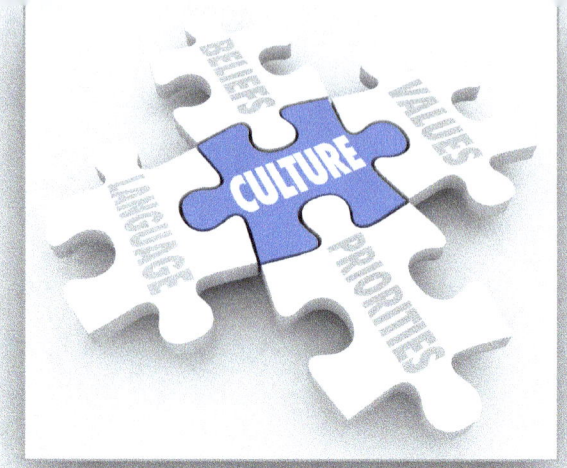

seems to be a consensus. Given those differences in circumstance, the results could be positive, from 15% to 70%, which is incredibly remarkable. We seem to be creatures dependent upon external validation for what is true. That feature may work to our benefit in situations designed for our benefit, yet leaves us vulnerable to deception in following the crowd behind a harmful, or untrue idea.

Even though the 'pill', as it were, is fake (sugar pill), the results are real. In the case of pain, the greater the pain, the greater the relief. It was discovered afterwards that the brain of the subjects studied had produced endogenous analgesics which really did relieve the pain and the pill was the trigger. (Dr. Faith Brynie, *"The Placebo Effect - How it Works,"* Psychology Today, January 2012) Other studies have found changes in the brain stem, amygdala, spinal cord and nucleus accumbens region of the brain, with increased activity in receptors associated with the brain's opioids, in addition to increased dopamine levels. This proves that the body is listening and responding to how we, as the fulcrum, are organizing around our experiences even on a biochemical level.

There have been thousands of studies on placebos and it's a little surprising what some of the influencers are. For example, the color and size of the pill have a stronger effect, two works better than one, capsules work better than tablets, and an injection is more effective than a tablet. In case you were wondering if motivation was a factor, look at these results: In erectile cases, regardless of receiving a real pill, a placebo; whether the subjects knew it was a fake or not, in 100% of instances their erectile dysfunction improved. (Timothy Newman, *"Is the Placebo Effect Real?"* Medical News Today, September 2017)

Placebos are the most effective for chronic pain, anxiety, depression, and irritable bowel, but have also had a beneficial influence on symptoms of Parkinson's whereby the presence of dopamine increased in the striatum. Studies also show that sham surgeries are as effective as real ones for some knee and back surgeries. The body will alter itself in one way or another in several, almost inconceivable ways, according to our interpretations of reality. Nocebo effects can happen when the subjects are told to expect a negative outcome.

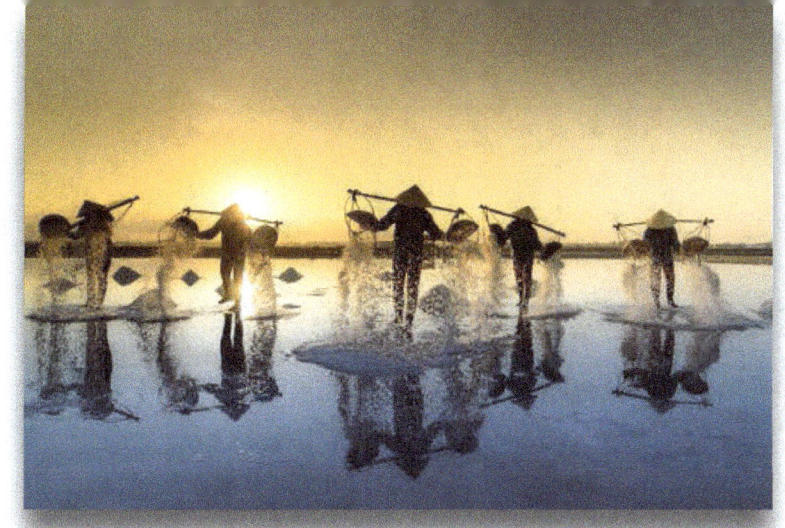

They are also effective when expectations are coming from the patient's doctor. Even with a sugar pill, if the doctor tells them that there may be unpleasant side effects, the patient's mind will produce those side-effects in their body. It shows that we are suggestible humans and that it can work both ways. Understanding a bit how the subconscious works in terms of suggestion enables us to not fall prey to how a great deal of marketing, sales, and even courtrooms work. Understanding it a little more enables us to learn how to program our own subconscious into having a wonderful childhood even though it may have never happened. What matters is what you and your system believe, and the results can be a heightened sense of health and well-being.

Belief is just part of what influences the reeducation of your nervous system. It will work in any case, but improvements will go more smoothly and quickly if you believe in the process. The body, for the most part, is honest; it acts according to what it's been told even if we forgot when it got the message. In that regard, in most cases we can't just talk ourselves out of a condition, an ache, or pain using the mind alone when subconscious emotions are part of the package. We'll need to address that original incident that has tied it into the system that way. Once either presence with awareness is clear as you move mindfully, or the anatomical structures involved are specifically tuned into as you move, the message will get through. The brain will reflect that clarity and specificity and update the body. You will feel the changes happening immediately.

There are several contributing factors to most patterns, and it will help to get a clearer idea which aspects of ourselves and our environment hold the patterns in place. One aspect is definitely our belief and expectation, along with how we feel about the source of the information we're believing in. For example, my mother believed that she shouldn't take medication for the high blood pressure that developed suddenly later in life, even though she found out that she'd developed atherosclerosis and phlebitis, as well as hardening and inflammation of the arteries. Her entire life she'd had low blood pressure, then it suddenly spiked.

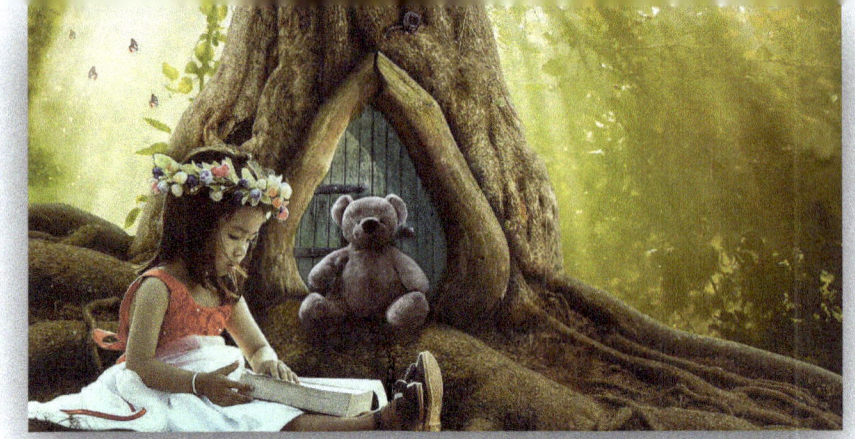

Her entire life she hadn't taken medication other than an occasional aspirin, and recently accepted that her thyroid was low and took medication for that. She decided to receive a faith healing from church for her blood pressure, and taking medication for it would mean that she didn't have faith. After experiencing six transient ischemic attacks in her brain, she still refused to take her medication. Speaking with her minister who was also her best friend, clarified the reason for her refusal, but it didn't help change the situation. When asked if she realized that she'd already had several strokes because of the high blood pressure my mother replied, "No I don't know that, but people have told me that."

Hiding meds in a milkshake worked for a while until she realized that it tasted a little funny and figured out why. I wonder why no one thought of better tasting medication for the elderly. In any case, it wasn't until her condition required a feeding tube due to her diminishing ability to swallow correctly, that we were able to consistently get her medication down, and by then offering her different types of nutrition through the tube had brought her blood pressure back down to normal. She refused to go against her religious beliefs no matter what it was costing her otherwise, and I had to respect that even if I felt sorry about the cost.

Some ingrained patterns have a great deal of significance and value to a person and will possibly not be changed. The decision for what the organizing principle will be for each of life's experiences is in the hands of each individual. We who care for them may need to share the weight of those beliefs and values. Nonetheless, retaining some sense of control and dignity in one's life when an elder becomes more incapacitated, is in itself a great value that deserves to be honored. In this case my mother and a community with shared beliefs expected her to receive a healing. It didn't happen in ways that seemed obvious, but I often wondered if her wish when she was younger came true: that she wanted to spend all day in bed.

It could be that her subconscious filed that wish and fulfilled it for her later in life. She'd worked so hard for so long, she also had a desire to be taken care of. Both of those wishes came true. Were there other unresolved issues that contributed to the plateau and limited response by her system? Probably so. Beliefs, although not

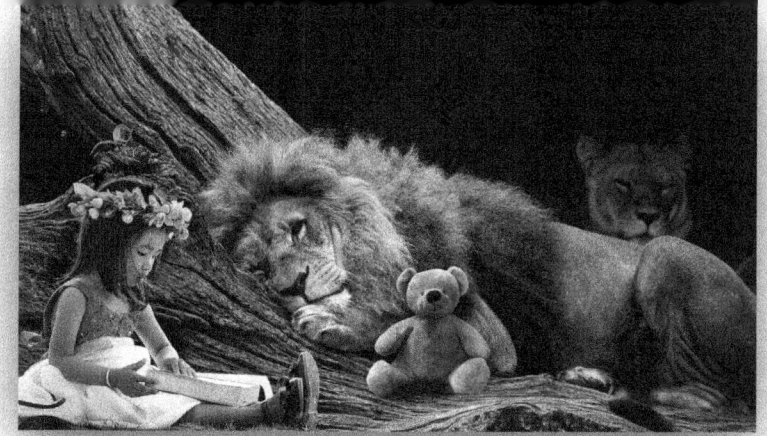

solid or tangible so-to-speak, tie us into a set of priorities that can at times be immovable. My mother did make a conscious decision at a critical choice point, and it may have been in service to her 'secret' desire to have deep rest with less responsibility. The "Be careful what you wish for," phrase may refer to the fact that your body and the Universe are always listening. Don't forget to fill in the details of what you want your wish to look like! When you or a loved one is moving toward changes in health status, it's very helpful to examine beliefs and to make efforts to become aware of subconscious impressions.

## Self-image

Another component that influences wanting to make changes that could be helpful in improving health and well-being is self-image. If the thing we want to try conflicts with the way we see ourselves, there could be immense resistance. The point of bringing up these possible hurdles to change is because the main obstructions fall into one action: making the dynamic decision. A dynamic decision has life force behind it in a way that propels you into action fueled by sincere motivation and a clear intention. A passive decision is a desire you file in your bucket list to do later, waiting for more time, more finances, a friend to do it with you, and so on. The intention is still sincere; more than a wish list, but taking action is not immediate.

A hurdle is a little obstacle (like getting a cast off), or series of events that need to pass before the timing is right, but an obstruction is more of a full-on roadblock that we may not even be aware of that is holding us back. That's the thing where you tell yourself, "I need to stretch more," but deep down you've only seen females go to yoga classes and it's not what a strong, virile male would do unless he's on the 'hunt'. Some may classify meditation and yoga in a "Kumbaya" type of activity that is too "touchy/feely" to suit their image. Females might avoid sports or sweaty exercise because it's just too 'yang' or aggressive; not befitting a lady's image or inclination. They may also feel like they're too weak; not realize their own strength.

There are two ways resistance can sit in a person's psyche: one is with charge and glue, and one is in a neutral way. Both ways can be subconscious. When you're

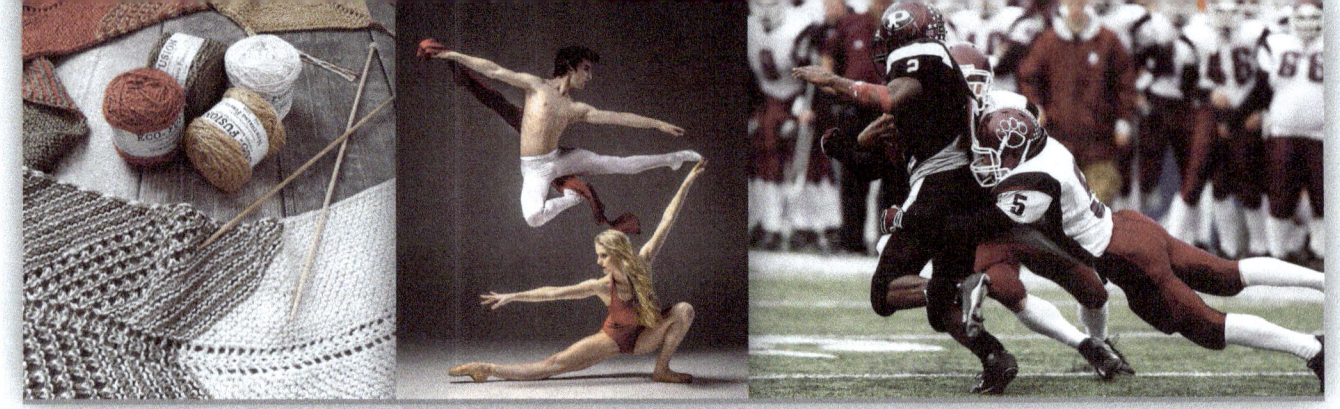

curious about why something isn't changing and light comes, for example, to an 'attitude' as being the reason, there are two ways that you may find yourself to be in relationship to it: identified and not identified. If you're not identified with an attitude that has charge and is pretty sticky in the way that you've been holding it, you can still let it go easily. Maybe just a little note to self, like, "Wow - I didn't realize I had that going on. Good to know, but I don't need it."

Rosie Grier gained notoriety as an NFL defensive lineman for the Giants and the Rams when he picked up needlepoint, traditionally a hobby for older women. Probably many people picked up the hobby after seeing Rosie do it. Tackle for the Pittsburgh Steeler, Steve McLendon, claimed that ballet is the hardest thing he's done. He joined the ranks of heavyweight champ Evander Holyfield and hockey's Ray Emery, who used ballet for cross-training to improve their performance. They didn't let their self-image of manhood get in the way of the wisdom that using your body in a completely different way opens up the possibilities of new ways the body recruits muscles to enhance agility, speed, flexibility, concentration, and balance.

A neutral stance in whatever you discover as being attitudes that are learned or inherited from society can tame the beast that would otherwise limit your life; sometimes in ways that can be unhealthy. My own self-image was a huge drawback in healing from a back injury because I wouldn't accept the fact that my ability to do many things had changed. I'd been fiercely independent and didn't want to ask for help in doing simple things, like in carrying something for me that only weighed one pound. I re-injured that disc over and over because I refused to accept limitations that my back needed just for a while in order to heal.

In the same way, I was determined to be a vegetarian due to spiritual and philosophical beliefs, even though it was part of the reason I injured my back in the first place. I'd grown up having meat at every meal; a diet filled with protein and a little veggies and potatoes on the side. Ignorance was part of this equation, because I didn't realize that people had different needs when it came to diet, and everyone I knew from a variety of backgrounds in our spiritual community was a vegetarian. I didn't see anyone else struggling with it knowingly. I didn't attribute the cause to lack of nutrition initially, but my joints were becoming more and more

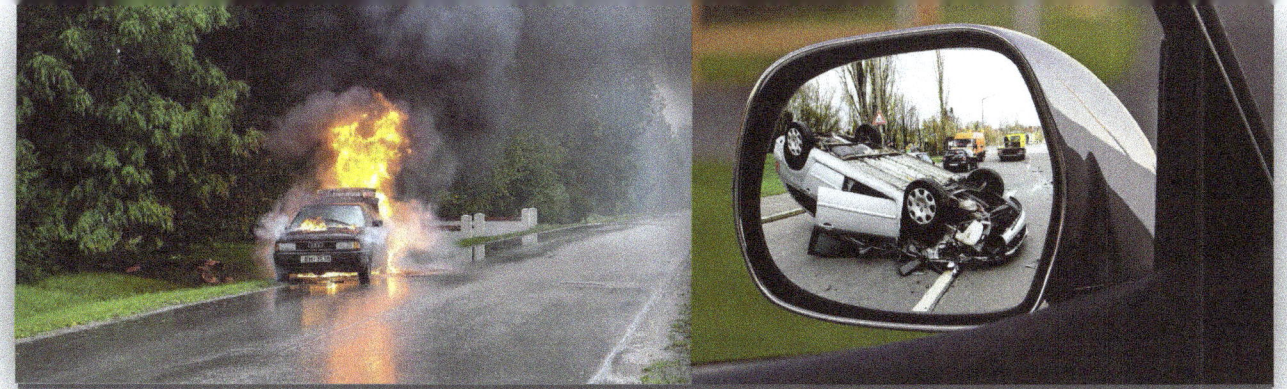

unstable, as were my hormones. Everyone in those days thought that rice and beans were a complete protein and would give your system everything it needed. It wasn't true for me, and by that time I couldn't even digest rice and beans. My system had also lost its ability to break down eggs, dairy, raw vegetables, and almost anything with a cell wall. My brain was getting super foggy, and my muscles were extremely weak, but meditation was easier, probably because I was in a daze half the time. It took several years of decline and being in constant pain before I was open to adding a different form of protein back into my diet.

Luckily, four years into the back issue I met Tom Hanna, started his training in Hanna Somatic Education, and in the first month was able to feel my body without pain again for a few moments. I didn't realize it at the time as I stood there on the sidewalk mesmerized by the lack of spasms, but I'd just discovered a calm, neutral zone in my body that was finally balanced. I remembered that felt-sense for the rest of my life. It became the gold standard for a baseline of resting tone in my muscles. From that sensory baseline I could discern changes in tension, which would then receive my full attention and immediate action. This was the beginning of a 25-year saga of putting out fires in my system that was filled with invaluable lessons in what I was doing to start them, or to keep them going.

My body felt like it had been totaled, with several systems in varying degrees of dysfunction. I'd finally found someone who held the keys to the missing link in my recovery from a physical point of view. That view was of utmost importance after years of intractable pain, so my motivation was really high in a dynamic way. Feeling a significant change in just a month validated that healing was possible, and that I was on the right track. My brain had also taken a hit due to lack of sleep and lack of nutrition, so it was also a struggle to kick the brain back into gear to study the information we were presented with in the course. It was the beginning of a long period of trial and error, of listening to the slightest warning sign from my system, and of beginning to be able to take responsibility for my role in my body's ability to heal. It had always done so automatically in the past so it took a minute for me to accept that things had drastically changed. That was an unrealistic expectation that had been difficult to shake.

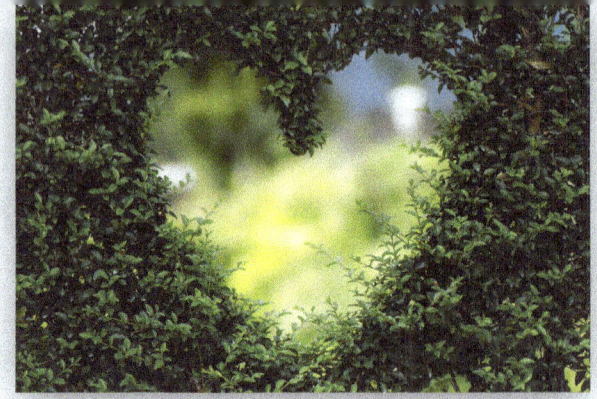

My digestion had been a mess, blood pressure was extremely low, blood sugar was also low, inflammation was chronic, my spine and sacrum were hyper-mobile, and with sleep deprivation being a regular occurrence, brain fog was constant. It's much more difficult to heal at a normal pace when several systems are so out of whack. The answer to the question of where to start was, for me, to keep the pain and inflammation down so I could sleep. If I could sleep, I could figure out how to balance the rest. As the fulcrum around which the changes were going to orient themselves, I was committed to being my body's ally and advocate. From that point on, I was fully invested in learning how to interpret the vocabulary my body used to communicate with me. From that point on, imbalance became my teacher.

## Modifying unrealistic expectations

There were many actions and positions my back wasn't ready for, but it was a huge leap in awareness for me to discover what it could do safely. I also learned to modify and expand the things that seemed to be on the 'no' list that turned them into a 'somewhat,' instead of a hard pass. My macho image had softened into a compassionate, caring one, willing to admit to the current fragile status. The somatic blindness was finally having its eyes opened onto a sensory field full of valuable information speaking a language I was then eager to listen to. Any painful departure from a neutral baseline, had me stop and ask my body how to modify what I was doing to make it okay. It might have been the length of time spent in an activity, whether I'd arched my back while bending, how far I'd bent over, etcetera.

I quickly learned that compressing and rotating on an injured disc exerted several pounds of pressure that produced immediate pain. I put this position on the 'no-no' list. This led me to avoid sitting down, even on my car seat. I'd lifted my pelvis by pressing my left foot against the floor of the car, and held my back against the backrest behind me. I stood to eat, to work at the computer, to talk on the phone, to watch television, and my work as a therapist and physical therapy assistant was already done standing. Eventually I could sit on a cushion with a donut hole to avoid pressure on the tailbone, but it took years before being able to sit on a hard surface again.

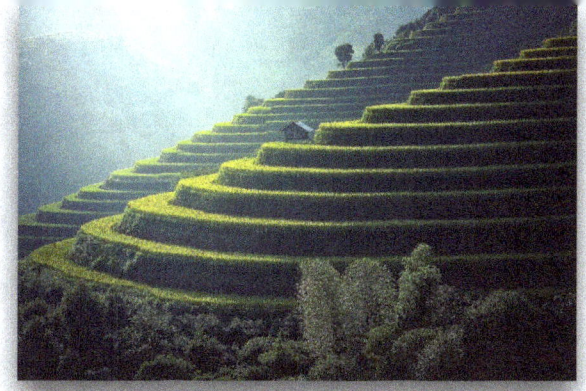

Like many people, nurturing myself wasn't an automatic response. It's a social expectation that you'd don't complain or baby yourself while you're injured. People who don't complain are praised; it represents strength in adversity, plus, no one wants to hear it. As a martial artist, we also shrugged off discomfort and pushed on. The way the macho expectation still showed itself was to rarely act like I was in pain. I strapped ice to my back when the hyper-mobile joints slipped out of place, then worked a 12-hour shift. Because it was often too painful to put weight on the right leg when the sacra-iliac joint was inflamed, I would hop up and down the stairs on the left leg. It never occurred to me to take a couple of days off when it was like that. I'd never seen anyone in my family take a sick day, and using sick days hadn't been a practice for many years.

Even though I felt reduced to a bowl of confetti that could be blown over on a windy day, there were limits to the extent I was willing to let it take my independence. I'd learned in the martial arts classes that we had an enormous amount of energy that was yet untapped. We'd practiced putting the energy of emotion into the task at hand so it could be transmuted and used. There were delicate, hairline choice points along these lines that needed modification. While I didn't want to completely give in to an orientation of weakness, I also didn't want to override the fragility of the healing process when there'd been tissue damage. Back injuries are invisible; they don't show like a broken bone, or a cut. People are a little surprised to hear that you're in pain and it even lends itself to folks thinking you're faking it.

In those days, back injuries were so common they were being called psychosomatic; a stress-based issue. There was even a book out at the time reporting that society had switched from getting ulcers to back pain once ulcers had become associated with stress. To be honest, a great deal of back pain is related to stress because chronic tension can tighten muscles in a painful way. It doesn't mean that chronic tension or strain won't develop into tissue damage. Degenerative disc issues, sciatica, arthritic changes, bulging or herniation of the disc can express in sudden or ongoing back pain. For that reason, it's good to find out what your particular case may be, because the treatment approach and exercises recommended would be very different if there's been structural changes. Many people already know what the status is, but if in doubt, do find out.

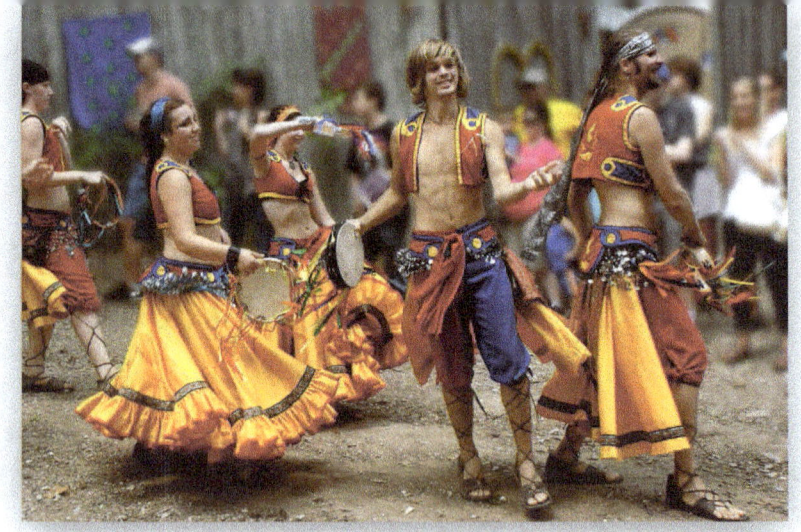

You don't want to be maintaining a brave face if there's real damage going on, because it could be getting worse in a way that will be difficult to remedy if you ignore it. Tens of millions of people experience back pain every year costing billions of dollars in treatment. Estimates are as high as 8 in 10 people admit to having this common type of pain in their lives. Lack of exercise is a common reason, but weight gain, kidney issues, infections, or wear and tear are also common causes. Even the most relaxed business setting doesn't expect to see or hear their staff in even a mild meltdown. Quite honestly, we didn't do it in my family either. No one really expects to hear or see emotional reactions to pain, but it's really important to use pain as a sign from your body that something's wrong.

This is another fine line that has to be tread, because the psyche is amenable to learning patterns just like the body is, yet a pattern of catharsis isn't healthy either. Society assumes that (invisible) physical and emotional pain are connected. It would be helpful to distinguish which is the case for you. Whichever is the case, the pain is real and needs to be dealt with before a serious condition develops. Some have found creative release in the arts, using dance, painting, acting, or music to express what they're feeling to help clear the charge.

A few of the somatic pioneers were looking for ways to wake up more feeling in the expression of music, in theater, or life in general, through their bodies. The culture of repression was having a stiffening, numbing impact throughout society. Leave it to the artistic types to inject a little more freedom of energy and expression into the world. François Delsarte, who had a tremendous influence that lasted through the ages, was a voice and acting instructor in the late 1800s. He'd experimented with ways for his students to create more fullness and emotional impact in what they expressed through their bodies. He began using postures, or poses to depict a certain mood, disposition, feeling, character trait, or quality. He was literally teaching them what emotional expression would look like in their bodies, if it were allowed to surface. A talented American actor, Steele McCay, brought the Delsarte method to the U.S. after studying with him in France.

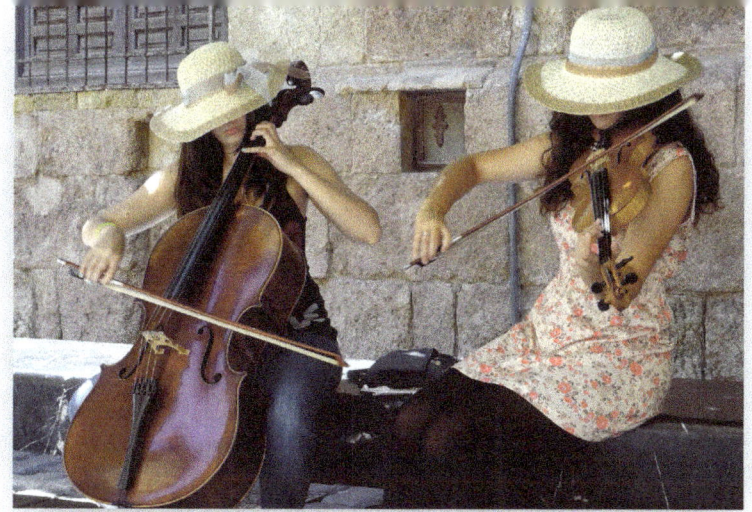

McCay's best student, Genevieve Stebbins had already developed her own work called 'Harmonic Gymnastics' when she agreed to teach the Delsarte method instead. Delsarte and Stebbins made a huge impression upon Isadora Duncan and a couple of dancers called Ted Shawn and Ruth St. Denis. The pair opened their own dance studio, started one of the first dance companies in the U.S. and later trained Martha Graham. St. Denis got some of her inspiration through dances from Japan, Egypt, and India. These women were part of a movement to find ways to be freer. They wanted to free their ways of moving, dressing, and even exercising in that era. They wanted a way to feel less confined and restricted in what it's supposed look like to be in a female body, particularly among the upper classes where Vaudeville was 'inappropriate'.

Heinrich Jacoby and Elsa Gindler paired up in the early 1900s for explorations in movement. These movements led to enhanced emotional expression in the music by the musicians' interpretation of the song, and also in their ability to connect with that music in their bodies. Connecting with your own body was such a key to regaining well-being around wartime in Europe. Gindler's personal 'experiments' led to remarkable reversals in health and mood through her ability to sense how she was using her body throughout the day. Capturing somatic snapshots throughout the day can be revelatory to how you might be subconsciously contributing to your symptoms.

Stebbins was also influenced by Gindler's work, called Gymnastik, whereby they both made long-lasting contributions to physical education, and the fields of exercise and gymnastics. The explorations of Moshe Feldenkrais were also influenced by Gindler's work, in addition to Gerda Alexander who coined the phrase, 'balanced tension' in the development of her work called, Eutony. Alexander Lowen, Wilhelm Reich, and Fritz Perls were all influenced by Gindler's sensory awareness practices, as was Charlotte Selver who brought Elsa's work to America. From here it began to take on more therapeutic aspects bringing versions of Somatic Psychology and Humanistic Psychology to the forefront of society.

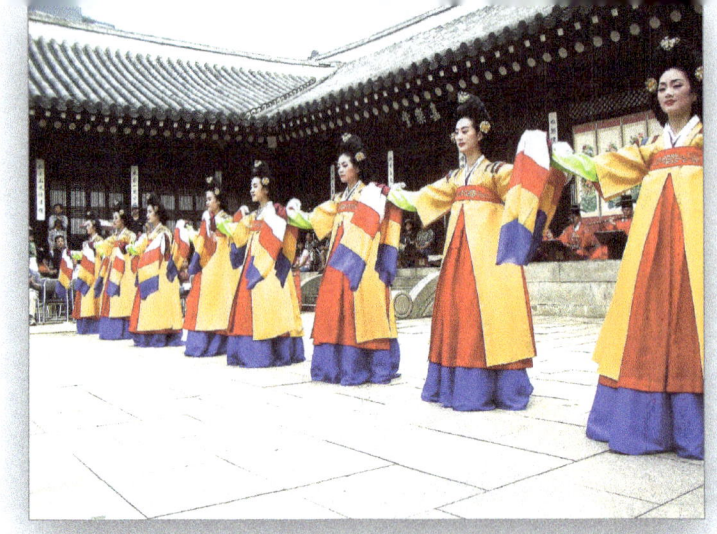

Gindler and Selver injected the field with the understanding that body, mind, and spirit are interconnected. Western approaches to physical and mental health began to take on transformative modifications, along with the enrichment of the performing arts as a result of their influences. There were spiritual injections in the approaches of St. Denis and Charlotte Selver who blended aspects of Taoism into her teachings, and it's been said that George Gurdjieff was Feldenkrais's biggest influence. Gurdjieff studied dances from all over the world but said that he was most influenced by the sacred temple dances in Asia, especially the Cham Dances of Tibetan Buddhism, and the Dervish dances of the Sufis. Apparently he believed, "that certain traditional dances were a form of sacred art whose purpose was to preserve and transmit esoteric knowledge and help to evoke an inner condition which is closer to a more conscious existence, or a state of unity, which can allow an opening to the conscious energy of the Self."

Gurdjieff, in his spiritual quest of twenty years through several countries, concluded that Universal wisdom of ancient traditions was passed down through music and dance. He wanted to teach many forms of movement, but reserved the sacred dance for his advanced students, emphasizing that in order to be successful, a commitment to developing 'presence' was needed. In many ways, the somatic pioneers in Europe were recapturing aspects of ancient movement and spiritual traditions which helped to enliven societies all across the world, as well as to improve well-being. In some areas and communities, the deeper work of seeking Universal wisdom is still being practiced, or being revealed, as in the case of several of the forefathers and mothers of Osteopathy. Diving deep into the body and the subtleties of its multi-dimensional nature will unveil infinite potentiality.

It could be that the long period of imperialism whereby local spiritual practices were squashed, left an unhealthy, disembodied by-product on all involved, including in the U.S. The world needed healing, and part of what was being discovered as being helpful, was regenerating spiritual roots. The other part of what was consistently found to be beneficial, was movement. Re-entering the body in a

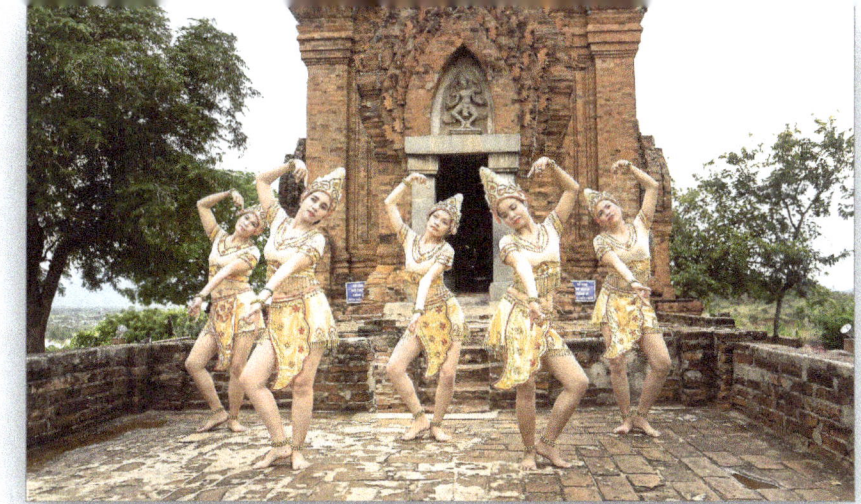

conscious, mindful way was helpful on many levels, even when healing wasn't the goal. Whatever the reasons for shutting down in the first place, the body is not attached to the circumstances that initiated the imbalances unless you are. Re-awaking the system can stimulate the body's own self-regulatory mechanisms at the same time you're waking up out of the trauma trance. Before some of those doors could reopen in my body, I needed to bring down the noise in my nervous system. The practice of sensory awareness and the concept of self-regulation taught me to discover which iterations of a movement could pass the pain inspector and which could not. I learned to live within accepted degrees of motion within a certain plane and wait for the body to agree when it was okay to expand those windows of okay-ness. Gradually extension, then side-bending, flexion, and last, rotation began to be acceptable. There were a surprising amount of dance moves that could live within those parameters, I'm happy to say!

First walking forwards and backwards in the pool, then sideways, then kicking on the side of the pool—all with a shorty wet suit on—became okay. In those days the temperature of the water could generate a spasm. The reward of honoring these boundaries was fewer and fewer days in spasm or pain, so each discovery was welcomed. It wasn't long before 10 minutes in the pool, and 10 minutes on the elliptical machine grew into 15 minutes each, then 20 minutes with 15 minutes of modified stretching. Baby steps was the name of the game. Shooting hoops was easier than racquetball at this stage, as was tennis, because there was less bending and sudden changing of direction. I even tossed in a little t'ai chi and chi kung which also needed modifications. Baby steps meant that the entire process of coming back to all these activities without modifications took about three years, which was also the length of the Somatics training.

Although my loose joints led to a sprained ankle before the training was completed, the new knowledge gained, and self-regulation explorations led to the ankle healing in a normal length of time. That meant that all of the systems were balancing and holding their balance—except the laxity of joints. This needed

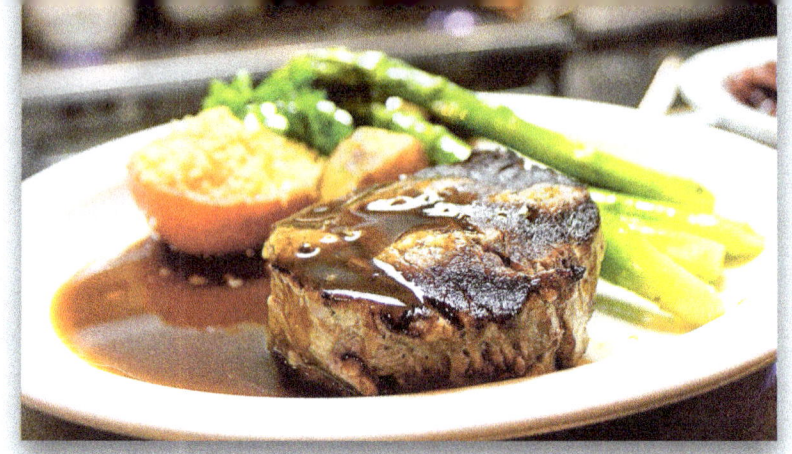

further exploration and questioning whether my diet now needed modifying in baby steps. It did. Adding fish and chicken made a big difference in the felt sense of solidity vs. fragility in my system, although it took a couple of months in each case before the nausea passed. I added enzymes and probiotics and before long, most foods were easily digested with the exception of dairy, avocados, Brewer's yeast, and eggs. The inclusion of TUDCA in my supplements gave my body what it needed to be able to process eggs again, which I was so happy about. I stuck to moderation, and the nausea disappeared. Avocados every now and then also worked out.

At some point along the way, after a few more injuries and the game-changing concussion, a neurologist insisted that I begin to eat red meat, which I did. There was a huge difference right away with no nausea and a big step up in mental clarity and overall strength. Adding meat had been recommended to me several times over the years, but the information out there was conflicted and it was all very new to me. I grew up eating everything with no problems, then suddenly I had to start all over again. I had a new body with different preferences. Part of my resistance came from the teaching that a vegetarian diet was more Sattvic—more refined energetically—which was needed to progress spiritually.

There was also a concern that negative karma was being created by eating the flesh of another animal, in addition to imbibing the creature's consciousness. Those were difficult precepts to overcome, as my spiritual journey was of utmost importance. My Native American ancestors had a reverent spiritual foundation, but also lived on buffalo and venison. This gave me some semblance of peace in the feeling that they weren't necessarily mutually exclusive. Food is medicine; it is a form of information and communication to the system in many, many ways and on many levels: for the brain, the mind, the hormones and nervous system, the microbiome, and internal organs, the glands, the bones, the fluid and excretory systems, energy systems, and pretty much everything we're made of. If there are toxins in the form of pesticides on the food you eat, the information delivery will be compromised in ways that are not healthy. When diet is determined by what our

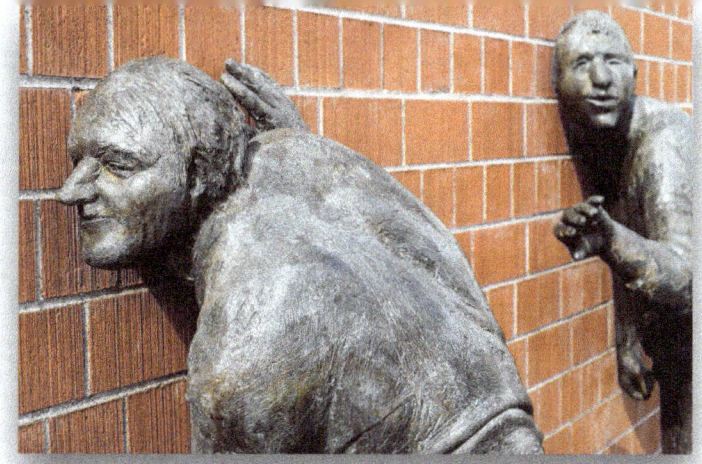

body tells us, instead of our habits, preferences, new books, or beliefs on the subject, another level of alignment with the body begins to happen.

Once the system is detoxed, rested, settled, and hydrated, there's a much better chance of what it tells us being accurate. I'd fasted regularly for 2 years before becoming a vegetarian, and did periodic intestinal cleansing throughout that period as well. Although it weakened me to the core, those 10 years as a meditating vegetarian that morphed unintentionally into being a vegan, was clarifying for my system. After that, I kept my inner ears open, and when my system gave me signals, I could trust those messages. I could also trust myself to make good choices, using moderation as a guide. Even after my digestive system healed, I continued to avoid grains, dairy, and soy. Lectins in general, but particularly eating chicken and turkey, could result in inflammation of the endothelium of blood vessels, which may have created the vascular issues with my mother. We'd grown up on a lot of poultry, which is supposed to be much more difficult to metabolize for our blood type, which is type B.

## Confronting medical muddiness

Medicine is an evolving science. There are new discoveries all the time, but it may take a while before the old information is deleted from common practice. That makes it even more compelling for you to stay on top of current studies on the subject of your concern. Doctors have become so specialized recently, that they don't keep up on recent findings outside of their field, and in general aren't up on nutrition or manual therapy options. Before you make a decision about which path to take, see if you can become aware of current beliefs you, your family, or your doctor may have in place. Do your own research before taking on their point of view. Things get a little muddy at times when we externalize doubts and assume others will disapprove if we do something outside of the norm. No one knows all of the facts in every situation, so it really helps if you know your body. It can help you to choose the best course of action.

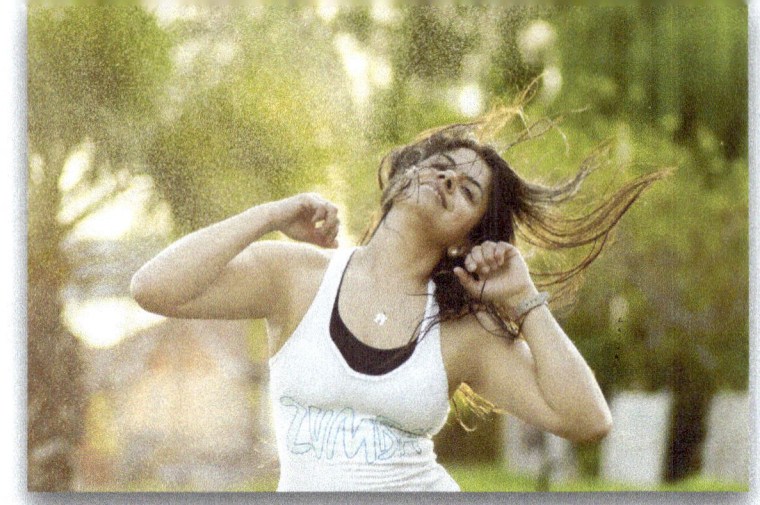

Most often the norm is the current standard of care by a medical authority. Case in point: although on one hand my mother wouldn't easily accept my alternative ideas about what would be best for her—with the exception for her religious beliefs—she readily accepted recommendations of her doctor without question. Even though I was standing up for her and getting her off of unnecessary meds, she didn't like me confronting or questioning her doctors, figuring they knew best when it came to medication. They didn't though, because they had her on at least six drugs that were inappropriate. I knew her, and was aware that her system hadn't changed that much in a few months. I realized that they were trying to contain symptoms using medication, and that they were already producing side effects.

Many in her generation did so even when side-effects were worse than the original issue, but there also were those who refused to go to the doctor. Our generation, the Baby Boomers, seemed to be the first en masse to question those authorities and become our own advocates. However, many of us are just as ignorant and innocent when going to the doctor, being totally unfamiliar with our bodies, with the new symptoms we're facing, and with the language the doctor is using to explain it. We are the most vulnerable to self-deception, or to giving ourselves over to an outside authority, when we're uninformed and out of touch with our bodies.

When I look back on how I viewed doctors and the medical community in the past, it looks pretty bleak. There was almost no information to go on. There was no Internet in those days, and no one was going to the library to look up symptoms to inform themselves. My family never mentioned physical issues or discussed them, as though there were options we should be aware of. If there was an issue we needed medical help for, we went to the doctor and did whatever they said to do and didn't question it. Alternative methods weren't really around in the '50s and '60s in our neighborhood so it was like staring into a huge vacuum.

Something began to break in the '70s when a surge of new information arose in the alternative medicine, spiritual, and humanistic psychology communities, and a huge awakening began to happen. Word spread like wildfire and many Baby

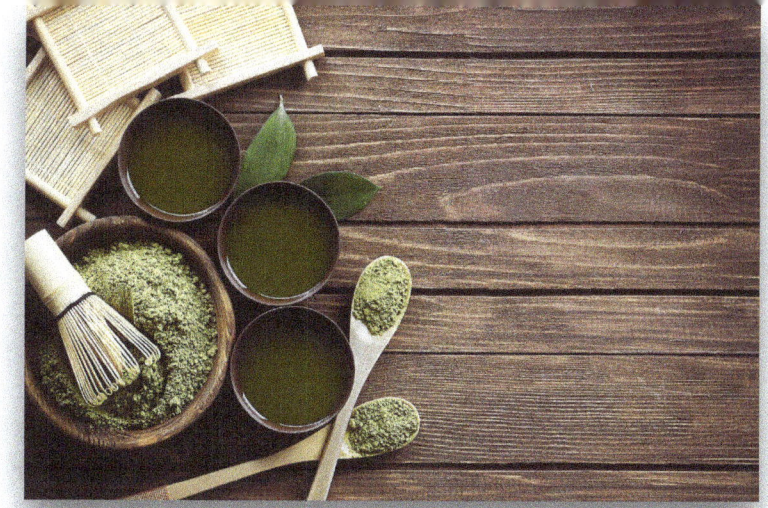

Boomers were gobbling up the new approaches with enthusiasm. That is to say that part of what can happen in the process of becoming your own advocate is empowering yourself to do so, even and especially in the face of the unknown. The concept may not land automatically in your awareness. Watching the behavior of family, friends, co-workers, neighbors, or even getting a whiff of it online through a podcast or webinar can start the wheels rolling in that direction. Sometimes we can follow old patterns simply because we haven't been exposed to anything else and aren't aware that another option is available. We check to see who else is trying it. It can be a gradual process of the new input landing on a fresh foundation of knowledge, or you can just take a big leap of faith and dive into something that sounds right or makes sense, even if you haven't heard of it before.

I'd worked for physical therapists and chiropractors for seven years and became pretty familiar with what they offered. I tried them both, as well as acupuncture for the back condition that developed, and found that within each of them I had a significant role to play as the middleman to discern which part of the treatment needed to be modified, edited, or deleted. It really depended upon which approach was being used, which modality within that approach, and how my system was doing at the time. It never worked to use the same approach every time. There was a time with a particular acupuncturist that the result was amazing, and another time or two that symptoms were exacerbated; the same was true for chiropractic work.

There are stages to the repair process and layers within those stages. It takes patience and kid gloves, and if given with care, even during exercise, progress can be much faster. Retaining conscious awareness after functionality returns will be a huge help in avoiding those compensations that lead to wear and tear. I've had hundreds of clients who have ankles that are still swollen from sprains that happened decades earlier. It never occurred to them to do anything about it once they could walk again without pain. Doctors tell them that ice only works during the first 24 hours, which isn't true. I still hear of people today who suffer tremendously due to lack of information about options. As the years pile on, so do the layers that get strung into the instrument that you'll be wanting to bring into a symphony of wholeness once again.

It's the aim of writing this book to unpack those layers and aspects of what may hang us up that, once you become aware of them, can be overcome quickly. Very often all that's needed is a decision, but it helps to have the data you need to make an informed decision. Some of that data comes from your body's vocabulary. Remember, only the pain is spoken in a loud voice, most of the body's vocabulary happens in a delicate whisper. Just like the somatic pioneers who vastly expanded and improved their somatic language through multinational inspirations, so can we learn and improve tremendously by opening up diversity in the potential languages we can converse in with our bodies. When what you're dealing with is brand new to you, or hidden in the subconscious, it can feel paralyzing to know which steps to take even if you feel motivated to take action.

Moving your body in gentle, conscious ways can access every part of where things may be sitting in your subconscious. It's simple, direct, and inexpensive. You just have to ask yourself if you want to go that extra mile for yourself. Feeling better is quicker and easier, so we'll often: go get a drink, take a pill to lift us up or to help us sleep, take a pill to shut out the pain, go for a run or have sex to discharge stress, overeat, strap ice on (like I did) and push ahead. One popular line I've heard countless times is, "I've got a high tolerance for pain," or, "I know I need to take better care of myself, but I've just been putting it off."

There are many reasons why people procrastinate, or flat out avoid making decisions to take care of themselves; some obvious, and some subconscious. If you hear yourself say it out loud, it might prove to be opposite of what you really want. For example, if you say to yourself, "I'm intentionally making the decision to continue having more pain and stress than necessary because _____", or, "The real reason I haven't made that appointment yet is _____". Once you admit it out loud, do you still feel the same way?

Maybe your actions and desires haven't been aligned; maybe you weren't aware that you hadn't made taking care of yourself a priority, as if you didn't matter enough to do so. Maybe you weren't aware of the consequences of postponing , or preferred to not think about them. The next chapter will go into more detail as to why folks let their subconscious decide for them. It's difficult to know what to expect or how to proceed in a vacuum, so I hope I can fill in a few more blanks for you. In any case, it's helpful to have high expectations of yourself and your body, because both are capable of great things.

# Chapter 3

# Making Decisions Conscious

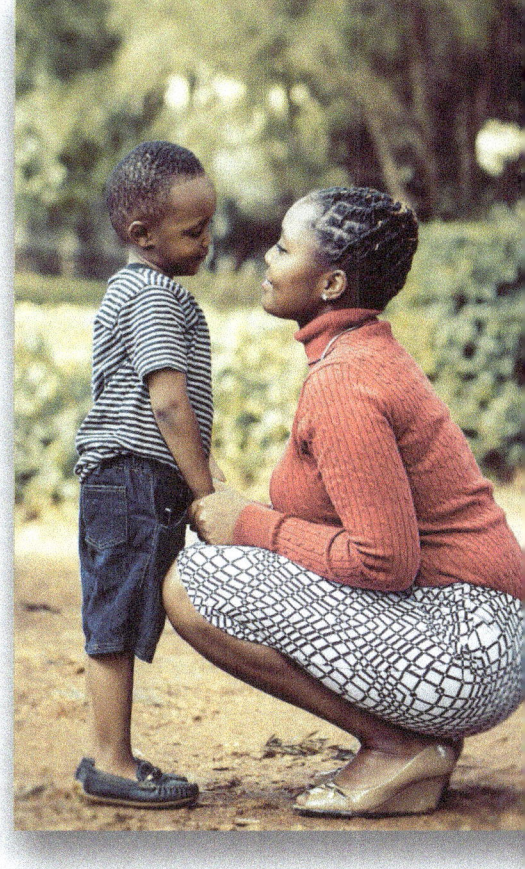

We've talked about many contributors to the decision-making process, most of which are subconscious. Without questioning where those deciding factors or patterns arose from, it's easy to become fixed into a whirlwind that could take you any number of places. It's like getting into a car with a taxi driver and not giving him an address. One of the factors that will be the most helpful partner moving through life with you is your awareness of your body. You become the mother to yourself as well as the compassionate listener to what your system is relaying to you as current status.

There is no expectation that the status will remain the same from day-to-day because you know how fluid living systems are, so you know to check in on a regular basis. So much of what motivates people comes from the desire to control life's uncertainties. Giving up awareness of what's going on in your body and mind is the surest way to lose control of your life. Getting in touch with your body and mind and developing an understanding of how they function is your best way to have some say over your destiny.

Awakening awareness is a vast task, literally, filled with wonderful revelations that can be limitless and invaluable. As alluded to in the previous chapter, so often in life we are in the position of needing to make a decision with very little background on the subject, and very little experience to draw upon. Medical conditions can be scary and have you facing into the unknown on more than one front. It can be helpful to talk to a variety of people who've been in similar situations. Ask what worked for them that might be outside of the traditional standard of care in modern medicine, as well as within it. You will likely have more choices than you know.

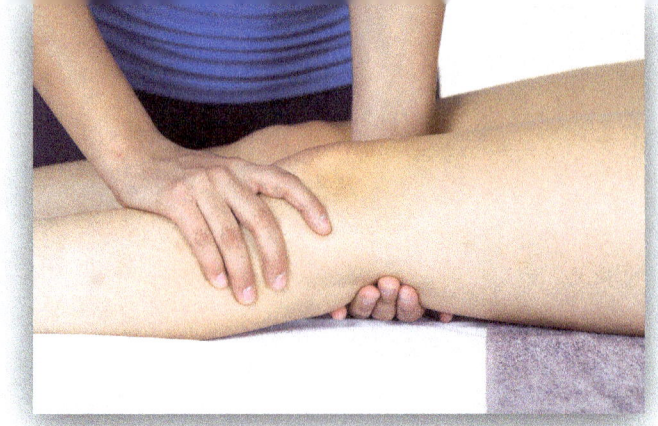

Whatever it is, surgery can always be an option as a last resort. Unless it's clear that there's imminent danger without an immediate operation, why not check out less intrusive options first? While I was working at a sports medicine and physical therapy clinic, a woman came in who'd had the scalene muscles removed on one side of her neck. I'd never heard of such a thing and couldn't resist asking her what happened. It turned out that she was an avid swimmer and had only been breathing from one side, locking up her neck muscles on that side.

Here's a situation where it seems like there may have been other options to try first, but it was too late. I wasn't aware of her decision-making process, but often use it as an example of a possible case where someone may not have investigated all of her options first. She only went to an orthopedic surgeon for suggestions on how to deal with the spasm and resulting thoracic outlet syndrome (restricted blood or nerve flow under the collar bone), and surgeons tend to recommend surgery. Be prepared for that going in; that recommendations will generally be made that are within the specialty of the professional you went to see.

I am certainly happy to refer to other professionals when I see a condition that's outside of my scope of practice, and it might be a good idea to ask for a referral if your current practitioner won't be able to resolve your condition. This was in the 1990s, and I believe folks are more pro-active these days and do their own research before agreeing to surgery. I've also spoken with clients who have had surgery recommended but are pursuing all other possibilities first. Here are some of the issues I've seen in clients and myself that impact how, when, and why decisions are made.

## Subconscious factors in making decisions

**The Unknown** - Fear of the unknown is real. So many decisions are made that attempt to make us feel more secure, more in control. If you're out of touch with your body, new sensations will bring up that fear. It's easy to feel overwhelmed with a novel physical symptom that's been causing daily discomfort. If it's brand new, you probably won't know what to do, and may not know who to ask. However, if

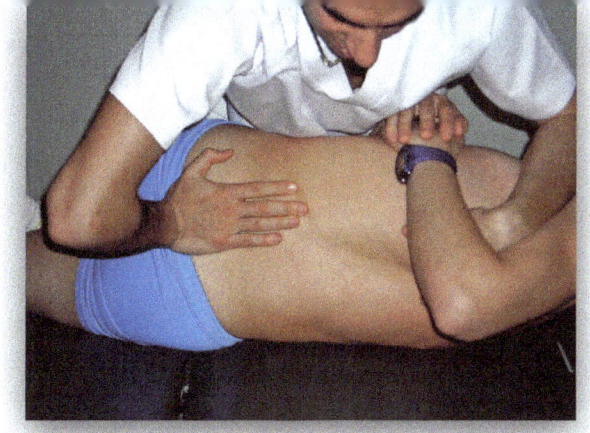

you do nothing, it can become so much worse that you're at wit's end. One possible solution is to not wait inside discomfort until you're at wit's end to seek help. It's harder to make the right decision when you're afraid and desperate. At that point you just want relief. I encourage people to start looking for answers at the first sign of imbalance, the first twinge, or some tightness that isn't letting up, nerve pain, numbness or tingling, before it becomes a chronic pattern.

It's helpful to be aware that by the time serious symptoms appear, the situation is likely so multifaceted that one approach won't be able to resolve them. It's also recommended that you include a manual therapist, someone who will treat your body using physical, hands-on methods, if the symptoms are physical. Even things like blood pressure and internal organ imbalances can often be served without medication if you get in there soon enough to discharge stress, or by checking in with an herbalist or nutritionist. Chiropractors use the concept of freeing nerve roots that innervate the organs and muscle to help the system make corrections on its own, and can be very useful. They are often expanding their methods to more holistic approaches these days, but I've seldom had an injury that could be resolved by chiropractic alone.

There have also been times when this type of treatment exacerbated the injury, had caused sciatica, and even caused a bulged a disc. High velocity techniques work for some physiques, but not all. If you're hyper-mobile or extremely stiff it may not be the best time to try that approach. It's helpful to ask on the phone or check the practitioner's website first to see if it's the right fit for you. It's also not a good idea to go for adjustments regularly, as your body can become dependent and forget how to self-regulate, even though the reasoning is to re-educate your system using repetitive treatments. For some it can irritate if not inflame the connective tissue with visits that are two or three times a week. That being said, these days chiropractors also employ cold laser methods, micro-neural current, ultrasound, and some also use massage therapists.

They are also usually equipped to take x-rays. If there's a firm, limiting restriction, it's advisable to get an x-ray first, and possibly an MRI to rule out soft tissue damage. Structural changes will alter the route of care. Physical therapy usually

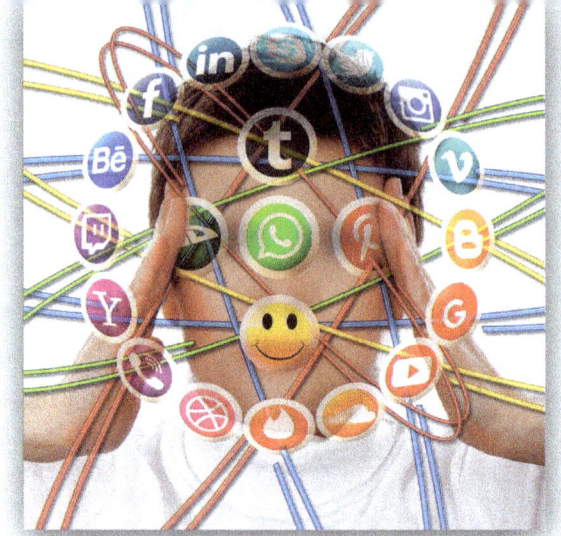

has a variety of methods to apply to an injury, including ice, ultrasound, phonophoresis, traction, electrical stimulation, massage therapy, and exercise. At times the physical therapist is also versed in myofascial methods, cryotherapy, hydrotherapy, kinesio tape, muscle energy, or other manual therapy practices that can treat nerve impingement. There are some who've taken visceral manipulation, pelvic bowl, or even a Feldenkrais training. Physical therapists are required to have continuing education to keep their license current, which is a good thing.

Again, you'd have to check their website or speak to someone in the clinic to give you a broader understanding of all the ways their therapists function for their patients. Along the way I learned to just cold call offices and even an advice nurse when I was completely in the dark about what my body was experiencing. Sometimes it's helpful to bounce something off of a professional to get their take on it, and to have help assessing whether it's an emergency type of thing that I shouldn't take chances with. There are situations that get worse with time, while others improve. Once you know your system a little better, you'll be able to tell if it's the type of thing you can 'wait and see' with to let time assist in making the determination. For example, sudden swelling is generally something not to postpone getting help with, but you can also get advice on how serious it might be.

One time an angry yellow jacket bit me in the arm after I wouldn't share my orange juice with him, and that evening my arm began to get red and swell quite a bit. This was brand new, but I wasn't sure if it would go away on its own or continue to get worse and spread. I called an advice nurse, then a Chinese doctor. The Chinese doctor said that he knew of a traditional remedy taught to him by his grandmother, which was ammonia. He went on to say that the purest form of ammonia was mid-stream urine, and to try putting some on the affected area. I followed his advice and the symptoms immediately began to fade and resolve.

In another instance my joints began to swell after taking an antibiotic, and I called the prescribing physician to inquire what to do. He told me to stop taking it and to

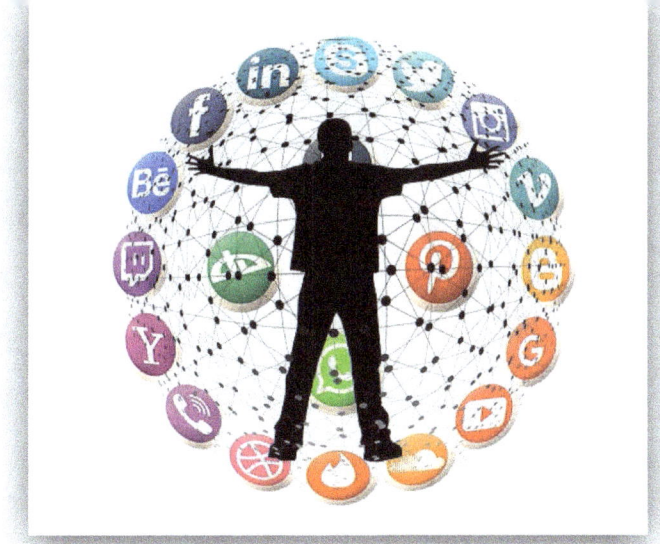

never take it again. I'm lucky I called right away to check. Apparently, I'm allergic to sulfa drugs. In a separate instance my adult daughter was helping watch over my invalid mother while I was out of town for the weekend when she called to say that my mother's thigh was swollen. I told her that thighs don't normally swell, so take her to the emergency room right away. Somehow, she had broken her femur above the knee. It healed beautifully in a normal amount of time with the aid of a few supplements for joint nutrition and bone broth.

A few weeks later, however, the thigh had swelling again. I called the physician's assistant to see if that was normal after such a long period of time, and he said that it wasn't and to bring her in right away for an ultrasound. This time it was deep vein thrombosis and blood thinners were required. Postponing that call could have cost her life. Many situations with the body are going to be novel, unexpected, and without a user's manual. Just because it doesn't produce pain right away doesn't mean it shouldn't be looked into right away. It's common to 'poo poo' new issues that don't interfere with carrying out daily life activities. Bring the unknown into the known by asking questions until you have the answers you need to take action.

**Time and money** - We'd like to think that new symptoms will go away by themselves, but there's always the chance that this time will be the one that will come back to bite you. If we don't let ideas of how strong and capable we are, or used to be, get in the way of making safer choices, it will save a lot of time, money, and grief in the end. Feeling like there isn't time to become involved in a series of treatments because you're too busy is a big gamble. The time it will take to correct if the conditions gets worse will be much longer, and more involved, so try to avoid that rationale if you can. Invest in yourself; health is absolutely the best investment you'll ever make! Certainly, if you don't have insurance and money is tight, you'll feel even more inclined to take the risk. Part of the unforeseen risk, however, is that what might have been a simpler, less costly solution will snowball into a more complicated, more expensive one if you wait.

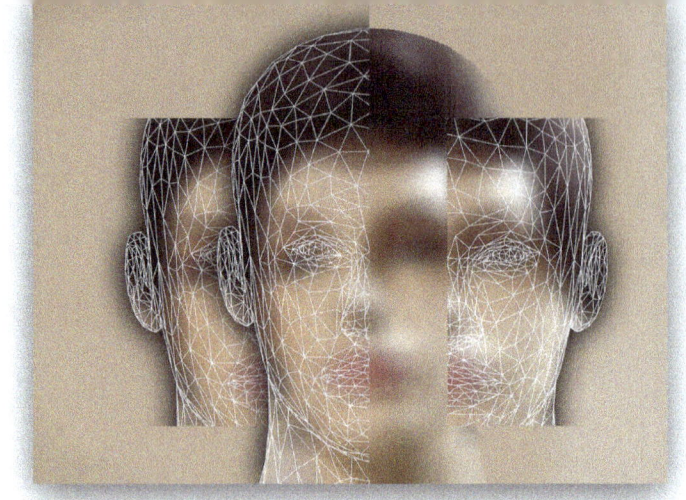

One silly decision I made to postpone had long term consequences. Who knows how this little stone got into a French fry that day? I bit into it and a corner of my tooth broke off. I kept going with my life for quite a while before it began to produce a little discomfort. When I went in to check it out, sure enough, a cavity had developed underneath the filling that was already in that tooth. It was at the point that a root canal and cap were needed. I couldn't see what was developing underneath, could still chew without pain, and didn't have much extra cash in those days. This was one of those 'wait-and-see' moments that didn't pan out so well. It turned out that the root canal was much more expensive than redoing the filling, but it went smoothly. The cap, on the other hand, did not.

It was fitted much too tightly and I waited too long to go in and complain about it. They changed the fit a bit but the pressure was still too much and it pushed the neighboring tooth out of alignment. Over the years, things really escalated and expensive braces were needed that caused many, many headaches. That lesson stayed with me and woke me up around the potential consequences of postponing. There's always a good chance that some unforeseen circumstance will open up a new source of income once you make the decision to get the care you thought you couldn't afford. Life often offers those happy surprises, and truth be told, I had to find the cash for the root canal, crown, and braces anyway.

**Stress** - Stress is a major determining factor for many of us. There are going to be times when you say in your head, "I just don't want to deal with this right now." Right away and without a second thought the situation is shifted to the back burner to simmer. When you already have so many things on your plate and feel like you don't have the bandwidth to entertain anything else, you're really squeezed between a rock and hard place. Either moving into a new challenge or avoiding it will be more stress. More often than not we opt to avoid confronting the new issue because we also have no clue as to how to deal with it.

However, things on the back burner take up energy and inner resources that can keep you up at night and create additional tension that may cause secondary

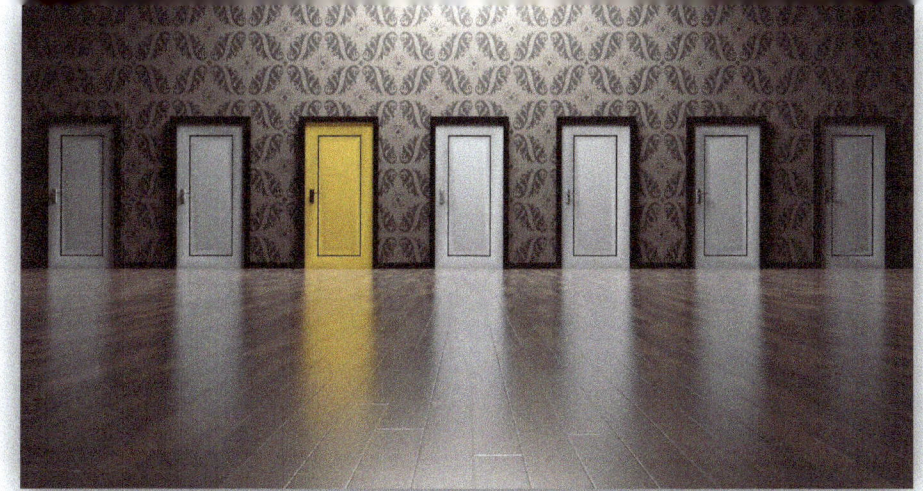

fallout. There are a few ways to juggle these types of situations without dropping the ball. Even sticky situations can include ways to address the situation before you make a decision. Consider taking a moment to tell yourself, "I'm going to make a call today to get more clarity on this issue. I'll ask who to see if I have these symptoms." Making this simple step does a lot to decrease the tension around the issue by bringing it more into focus, and by knowing which action to take.

Especially in times of stress it's really helpful to take a pause and really give the situation your best brainstorming cap. You'll find that a good idea is waiting to happen that will only require about 5 minutes of your time. It's so easy to skim over situations when stress is already present, or when things are moving so fast you can't quite catch all the details and implications. There's no better time for self-care. I began looking into ways to mitigate stress in my body with adaptogens. I discovered that the brain and adrenals would be less fatigued by using herbs or teas to help reduce cortisol levels. Astragalus, Ashwagandha, Vitamin C, as well as Tulsi, Lavender or Chamomile tea were all helpful.

Essential oils can also be a wonderful remedy for stress, as they have properties that are medicinal, researched, and effective. Lavender is the most popular, but Geranium, Ylang Ylang, Marjoram, Rosemary, Lemon Balm, Greenheart, Agarwood, Cedar, and Palo Santo are very helpful as well. Diffusing them through aromatherapy, dropping some in a Dead Sea Salt bath, and mixing them into the lotion I use after a shower are my favorites. Essential oils are also uplifting and calming, and contain several beneficial organic compounds to decrease inflammation and enhance the immune system. I needed to let my system know that I was paying attention, taking care of the workload, and of myself.

One healthy choice I made was to always tell myself the truth about how I felt even if the emotion itself wasn't expressed. It's fine to put on a happy face at work when you don't feel your best, but it's better to be honest about it so that your body isn't conflicted. You can say to yourself, "I wish I didn't have to go in today, but it will be over soon, I'll meet some lovely people, and can return home soon to rest." This

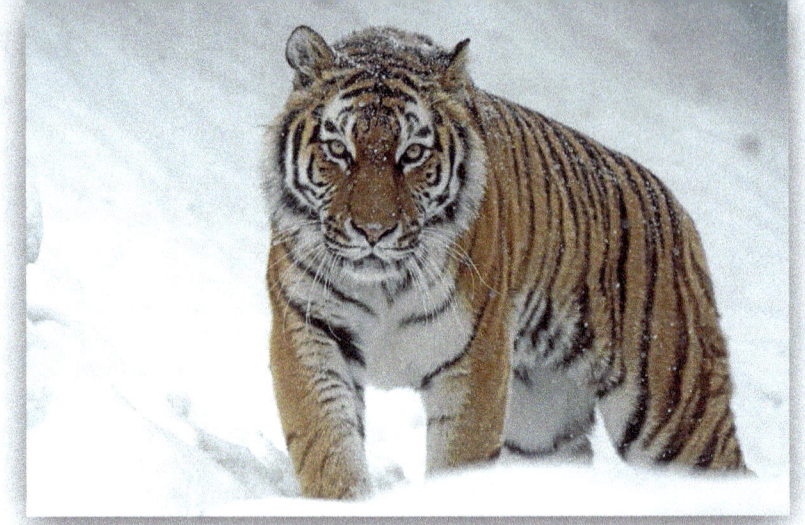

way your body and heart know that you received their messages, are present for the issue, and are listening internally so that you don't overdo it. Not all feelings are immediately actionable, but when you have a clear plan to take care right after responsibilities have been handled, your mood is lighter, your body cooperates more with the tasks at hand, and you have something to look forward to.

Having an open conversation with my body and myself gave a sense of closure to each day's activities that was in itself a great stress reducer. It acknowledges rather than represses feelings. I've seen many clients and friends who have wonderful, upbeat, personalities fall with health issues like cancer, asthma, MS, and other major conditions. They'd often had unresolved childhood abuses stored beneath emotional burnout or job stress as an adult. Since the same fate took many family members early on in their lives, I wanted to keep all the subconscious closets cleaned out and pay attention when current issues triggered new hiding places. Of course, exercise in moderation that includes cardio was always a help, but that's in the category of 'feeling better,' not in the category of healing.

In addition to the review each year of, "Am I aligned with my life purpose, and is there anything that needs to be added, adjusted, or removed?", I began checking in daily to ask the same questions. I asked if there was anything I could've improved upon in any interaction I'd had during the day. If there was, I made a plan of action, along with when to carry it out. That turned out to be a wonderful practice! There did come a point when I also promised to end the pattern of using every ounce of my energy to the point of depletion, and to work at a pace that suited the energy that was actually available and not more.

**Fear** - Pain can often be scary, no doubt, and fear is a natural response to it when the source is uncertain, the intensity is overwhelming, and there's no end in sight. It happened to so many patients after a car accident left them unable to work, with bills that couldn't be paid while pain isn't subsiding, and the future looks bleak. Perceived helplessness in the midst of pain can lead to anxiety, especially when

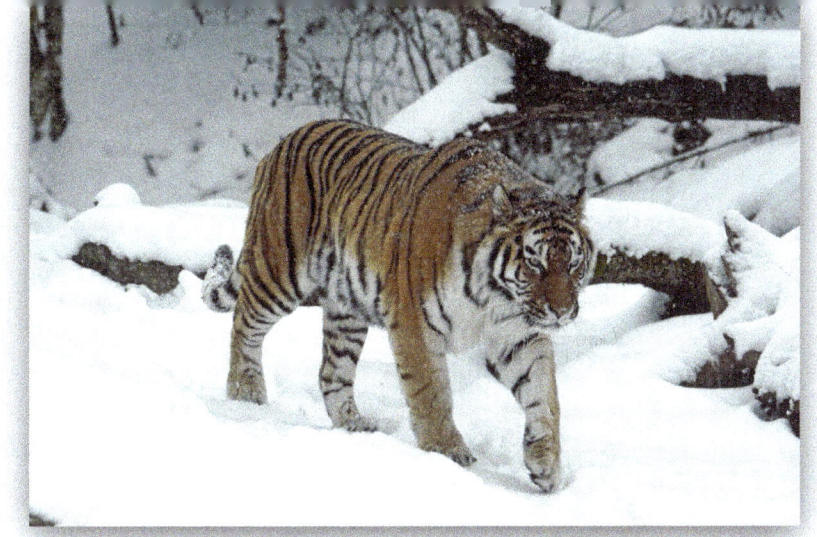

you don't know what to do to improve the situation. Fear can also become a type of denial whereby you pretend the unusual symptoms don't mean anything. You tell yourself it's no big deal, and you have a high tolerance for pain, waiting it out.

This was the case for my father who wouldn't go to the doctor when he had lung cancer. It had spread to his brain before family members insisted that he go. There may have also been some distrust, some fear of the unknown, or not knowing how to interpret the symptoms. Some folks would rather not know than face the worst-case scenario. It was also true in my case when I was in my 30s and I remained in a risky, fear-based denial, coupled with 'wait and see' because the doctor recommended a biopsy. Some hard object on the pillow woke me up early one morning, and when I lifted my head to see what it was, I discovered it was attached to my neck. There was a lump the size of a golf ball in there and it was sore.

I treated it like a toxic overload, and put some clay on it to see if it would pull the toxins out of it. I called my mother after my visit to the doctor to let her know in case my risky choice to refuse the biopsy didn't pan out. I wanted to drive across the country and wasn't going to let that stop me. She and her friends at church prayed for me and in a few days it was gone. I never knew why it came, but was grateful that it went. I didn't want my body or mind to bring it back in by thinking about it. Prayer is real; it's an appeal to the Higher Power to act as the fulcrum and reorganize whatever was appearing back into balance. The best case scenario is that you as awareness enliven your communion with your Higher Power and act as One in mediating imbalances.

Knowing that there are treatment options can reduce fear and prevent the consequences of avoidance. This is 'tethering your camel' in practical terms even as you pray. There are many types of fear or anxiety that could forestall a visit to get things checked out, including not wanting to hear what the medical professional has to say. Maybe my father didn't want anyone to tell him to stop smoking. Fear of loss of control, personal power, or of your independence shows itself in many

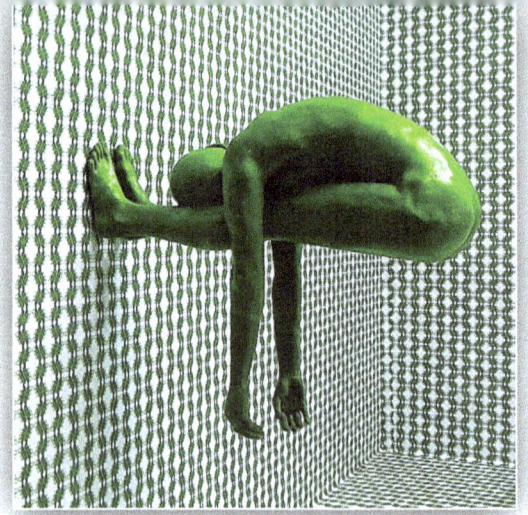

situations. Several people are afraid to get off of medications that aren't working because the side effects of the withdrawal are so intense and dangerous. Medications that create brain changes are particularly notorious for this.

One client was told she might enter a catatonic state if she stopped taking the antidepressant she was on that was actually making her more depressed. Self-sensing forestalls becoming dependent upon outside authorities who may not have all of the answers for you. Prevention is far superior to negotiating the territory of side-effects and withdrawal issues from pharmaceuticals. Looking for an easy way to feel better often winds up as an addiction that makes you feel worse down the road. Tied in to these types of resistance can be fear of change. There is a widespread belief that people don't change for a reason; many prefer not to. It does require a degree of focus and desire while the nervous system creates new pathways. That process creates many unfamiliar sensations while the new learning establishes itself against old backdrops, and a type of uncomfortable insecurity can result. The insecurity of unfamiliarity is unsettling.

People resist that feeling of uncertainty and insecurity with a passion, and attempt to use distractions to occupy the mind and avoid the issue. Routine hides the uncertainty of life from us, hence the resistance to break from the comfort of routine. Realizing that the discomfort is just a sensation during the transition to a new experience can help it be less scary. It can transform fear into excitement. Failing health is one of the main precursors to the step where their individual freedoms are taken away; where a sense of powerlessness intrudes. That discomfort is coupled with the fear of losing your favorite activities. There have been so many horror stories about folks getting worse after treatment. How do you choose the best one?

Most of my friends who have needed surgery send out a request for prayers on social media to help deal with the fear; and the same is true for cancer treatments. In so many ways we fear for our life; for life as we've come to know it. Fear bypasses the logical part of the mind and brain centers, so it needs you to be

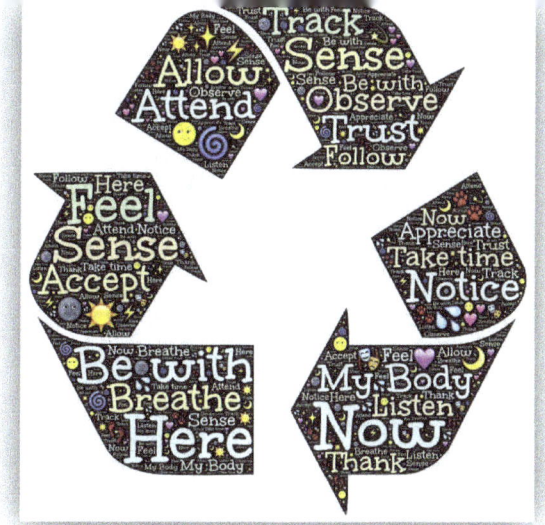

present as the superior officer so you don't identify with it and create stress chemistry. The irony is that avoiding decisions that could save your life due to the fear that you might lose your life, or lose control of your life, is itself paralyzing. Fear of death is under the same category as the fear of the unknown. A huge inescapable unknown is the future. Outcomes are difficult to know in advance, but you can remember that there are many, many options to improve the situation that you are currently in that you don't know about yet. The gift in many catastrophic injuries or illnesses is that you learn to live in the moment.

You as the fulcrum, are the most direct way to overcome this emotion. When fear becomes an object in awareness; a bundle of biochemistry in your body instead of who you are, you're free. Free as a being, and free to make a clear, informed decision. To help your fear reaction abate, you can ask yourself, "What exactly am I afraid of, in a sentence or two?" Most people know right away and can voice it, but haven't proclaimed it aloud. When fear remains in the back of the brain instead of the front of the brain, it seems much more powerful than it really is. When the answer to your question surfaces, It may be something wildly unrelated to the actual situation, or something irrational and simple, as most fears are. One way to settle the uncertainty is to call a healthcare practitioner and get the details of what the visit would entail.

Prepare yourself and your mind for what to expect. Reassure your mind that the solution can't arrive until you've identified the problem. Remind the irrational part of your brain that the healthcare practitioner isn't going to kill or torture you, and will instead be the first step in feeling much better. One stress remedy recommended to me by my spiritual teacher freaked me out. The first time I scheduled a sensory deprivation tank—a big tub of water with no light, no sound, where you float in liquid that's the same temperature as your body—I panicked. I knew I was claustrophobic, but the space wasn't that small; I could stretch out. Nonetheless, I sat up in fear until I told myself, "Osho's guidance is always spot on. You know the ashram doesn't let people die during any kind of therapy session! Think about it.

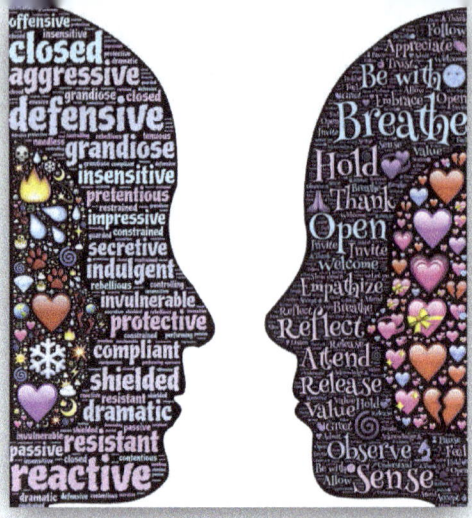

There's enough salt in the water that you can't possibly drown, and the attendant is right outside the door. You can call for help if you think you really need to. Now, please lie down and relax."

I had to laugh when I heard myself speak to the irrational fear out loud. The deprivation tank turned out to be one of the most exhilarating experiences of my life. My sensitized nervous system really needed it. I couldn't wait to do it again! Unless you're really in front of a major threat of danger, all fears are irrational. If you ask yourself what's really going on, that part of you will let you know and you can be the superior officer that calms the troops. If it involves another person, visualize yourself in the situation and come up with the best case scenario for your mind so it can feel prepared. Prepare your mind for the possibility that the conversation you dread won't go as well as you'd like, and let that be okay also.

Be ready and flexible for any response from the other person so you won't be anxious about it not being a particular way. Give the other person freedom to respond any way they will, knowing that they don't have to bend to your preferences in order for you to feel safe or comfortable. There's less anxiety when you strive to be in control of your own mind instead of another person's behavior. Very often we're afraid of what the other person will say, including the medical professional. If you let whatever it is be okay in advance, the fear will dissipate. Just know that you will handle it appropriately, whatever it is. It's natural to become a little on edge and defensive when you *feel like you don't have a defense* for the next issue you need to face. But you are your own protection.

Your presence and open mind is all the defense you'll ever need. You may have forgotten to trust yourself. Trusting in your ability to hear one new piece of information, and ask questions about a few options to resolve it is enough of a first step. Once you've calmed down your mind, the body will follow pretty easily. If you hold steady in the place of reassurance with your body, taking a few slow belly breaths, holding your chest up high with shoulders down signaling all is fine, your body's chemistry will also begin to shift. You can sing, chant, get a massage, do

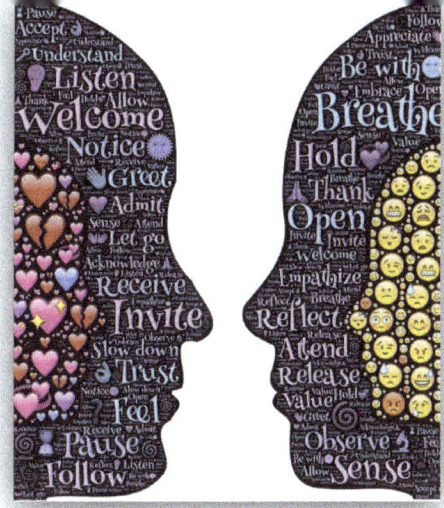

some conscious movement, meditate, take a walk in nature, and give your body several cues that let it know there is no threat. The stress chemistry will dissipate. Body chemistry is not the boss, you are. Conscious movement, like having a conscious conversation with your body that leads to a conscious decision, settles the nervous system as it settles the mind.

Making fear a conscious process brings it out of the foggy shadows and into a form where you can see all the shapes and corners of it clearly so that it doesn't seem like a monster hiding in the dark that can overwhelm you at any moment. The simplest way to dissipate fear of the unknown or of loss, is acceptance of whichever outcome you most dread. Let it be okay. It immediately drains the power out of whatever you were attached to as an outcome if you let it go beforehand and give freedom to the outcome. Also accept the fact that you are capable of handling any outcome, even if you can't control it.

**Negative self-talk -** Whenever you take a step back from your thoughts and make it a practice to notice them before deciding to follow them, you might be in for a surprise. You may notice that there is a narrative running without you. It's not being generated by the superior officer. If the officer is following automatically generated thoughts, the troops are in trouble. Remember that thoughts and feelings that were impressed upon us often become stored internally. They have been learned from somewhere or someone and can be triggered by association in an automatic way. We as the fulcrum around which they are organized are the one who decides whether they are valuable, useful, or not. The brain and body are receivers, processors, and transmitters of all types of input. You may have internalized a narrative from anywhere; from television, peers, social media, parents, anywhere.

In my case it was usually something my body or mind was struggling with that triggered negative thoughts. I'd been telling myself defeating or discouraging things about paperwork for so long that it had become a recording that got downloaded and replayed unconsciously. I'd identified with the record and made it part of my personality as an 'opinion' or attitude. A big part of the reason I didn't like it was

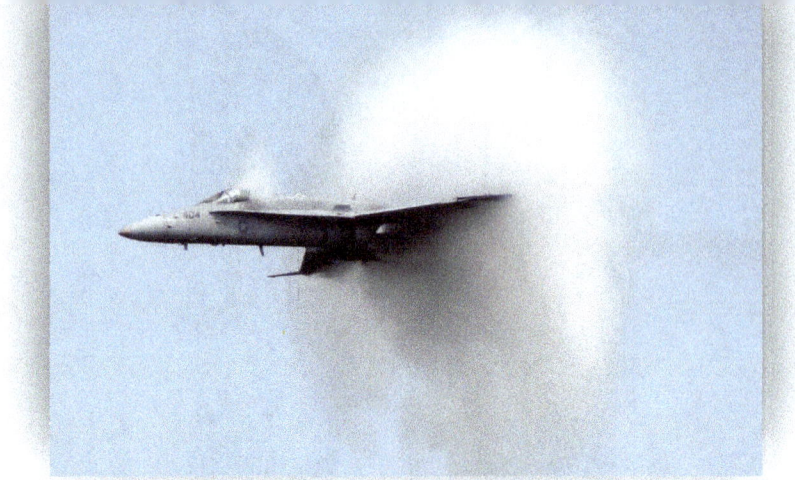

because I wasn't good at it and that sensation of being unsuccessful with it created an uncomfortable feeling inside my body. You could say that it literally got on my nerves. As a business owner, there were always so many forms to fill out that I didn't want to be strapped with a negative take on something that happened so often. I decided to at least take a neutral stance, engage with it in small doses, and shift activities when that uncomfortable sensation kicked in.

This was a low hanging fruit I could use to practice how to reduce negative self-talk. Paperwork can become an enormous struggle after head injuries, at times stimulating a few expletives, a sour attitude while doing it, and avoidance with consistent procrastination. Having ADD and dyslexia on and off made it almost impossible to focus and get it right. I couldn't change my brain right away, but figured that changing my approach to paperwork would make it easier for my brain to accept the inevitable. There was one main instance that helped me to reorient my attitude by example and re-associate the noxious elements of filling out or generating forms. I didn't want dislikes to be a major decision-maker for me.

I'd asked an employee to do something that in my mind, I assumed she'd agree to half-heartedly; like sweeping leaves from the walkways and parking lot. Hardly anyone wanted to do it. Instead she said, "I'd be happy to do that for you!" It was the most wonderful response I'd gotten from an employee about anything in a decade. It did something to my psyche that forever helped the approach to any type of distasteful task. What would it feel like inside if I said that about filling out a form? I tried it a few times, flipping the script into, "Oh good! I can knock some of this out now!" and it really did transform it. I began to feel good about completing a task rather than bad about having the task in the first place. It was a sonic boom level of breakthrough for me.

I could feel the reward chemistry kick in right away and change the climate of my initial resistance. I always feel a little lift inside by showing appreciation rather than disdain for any task. Being diplomatic with yourself helps tough tasks go down easier as a way of acknowledging and reconciling both the 'yes' and the 'no' inside.

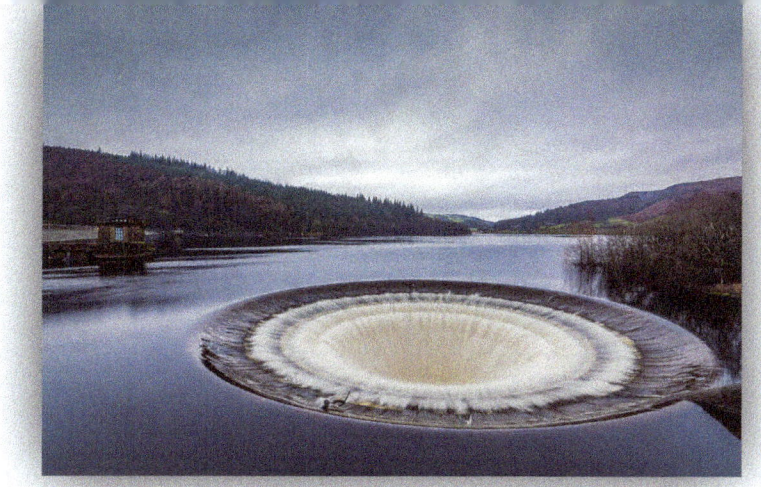

Arguing with yourself inside with what is basically like arguing with files in a cabinet. It's a perfect moment to see if some of those files can get rewritten or tossed out. Many of us received more blame than praise growing up, and it becomes a subconscious self-talk or sub-personality that we've internalized and believed as being real. Being aware that what we often hear inside as self-criticism is just some internal recording that's being activated frees you from its contents.

I felt free of the control that unsavory, unavoidable situations had over me. Pairing them with my favorite things, with an agreeable disposition towards them, took away their power. The same method can change the self-talk about going to the dentist, or doctor, or for any treatment you know you should get. We do function like Pavlov's dogs, so why not retrain the psyche in a favorable direction? The main thing was how these shifts made my brain feel, which changed the sensation in my nervous system and eliminated the negative thoughts. There are tons of ways that we run ourselves down, or run situations into the ground with negative feelings or attitudes about them. Remember that the brain and the body are neutral until told otherwise, and negative thoughts change the way that biochemistry works. They can just as easily create dysfunction and imbalance as a bad diet can. We do literally eat our words!

I use it to overcome resistance in getting myself to the gym. I just keep a focus on knowing how good it will feel afterwards. Negativity isn't our nature. It's a symptom of imbalance. There is also quite a bit of research out these days linking diet and the microbiome to mood swings, including anxiety and depression. These could also be sources of negative thoughts. Don't take it personally if your brain is putting out negative thoughts. Use it as a communication from your body that something is off. It may be a food allergy, hormonal imbalance, toxins building up, a low grade inflammatory process or infection. If you don't recognize the narrative as an old pattern, check some other sources of imbalance. It might be time to find a new job, or fix a personal conflict. Your body may be sending the message through thought patterns.

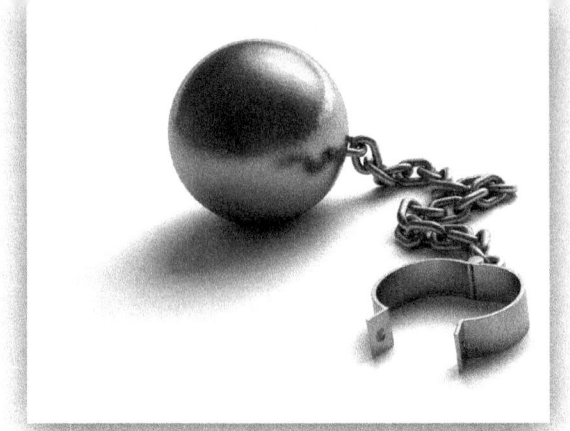

**Pressure** - There are many sources of pressure, all of which deserve respect for how they influence decisions. They are worthy of a deeper look so that we can check into the validity of the source, and whether it's real or imagined. External pressure in the form of deadlines and tough decisions that have high-risk consequences is real. Physicians, nurses, social workers, police officers, and even teachers have a high burnout rate. However, veterinarians' and construction workers' suicide rates have been on the rise and were already higher than the norm. They all have to deal with countless complex situations, often with complex people in the midst of many aspects that are out of their control. Jobs that have 'failure' built into them, like veterinarians who have to euthanize animals that could have been saved, are vulnerable to ongoing strain.

Substance abuse is often a way of coping with stress and depression, and suicide is put on the table as a way out of the pressure. Internal pressure often comes from external circumstances that are difficult, or that seem impossible to navigate or control. Even rescue dogs were becoming depressed when they weren't able to find survivors in an earthquake or mudslide. Finding ways to make these situations rewarding so the brain doesn't crash is challenging, but not impossible. Inserting little moments throughout the situation that inject it with love and compassion, with meaningful ceremony, music, prayer, or with symbolism through mantras, yantras (special patterned images), are immensely helpful.

Self-inflicted pressure is usually due to internalized, high expectations that can't be met, but can also be from learned social imprints and prejudices. Society is filled with schisms and 'isms' that exert tensions with hyper-vigilance. Racism, sexism, ageism, political party-ism, discrimination due to religion and spiritual affinity, due to disability, title and social status, income level, size, intellect, or any other pecking order can puncture well-being. Humans are mammals, after all. The animal in us may be looking for power through a type of Alpha or Beta dog status in the pack. Using distinctions to put someone else down, by default raises our own perception of self-worth, especially if they think they've found justification. These types of pressures are often ongoing, so may be the type you try to ignore or avoid.

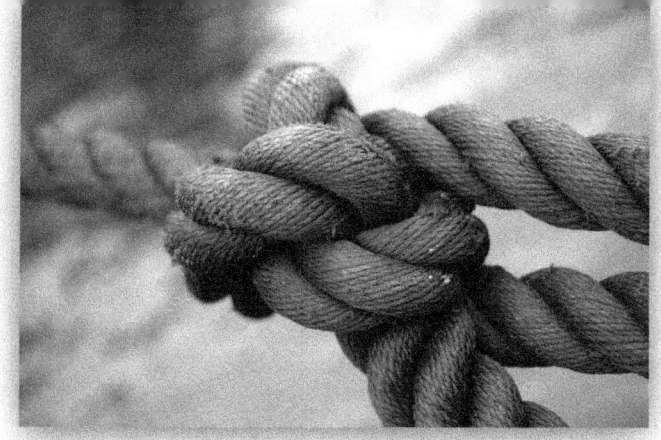

Your body would not be ignoring them. Your reactions to pressure are still alive in your system, but can be unlearned. Finding out if and where those stratifications may be living in your system could be very liberating, whichever side of the equation you find yourself on. Making these types of distinctions interfere with wholeness, due to the fact that separation is an illusion. It's like pitting one part of your body against another part, similar to how chronic stress or toxins create a confused autoimmune response. All living beings and living systems are interconnected, and just like a small physical imbalance can impact the entire system, a small social imbalance can impact the entire society. Taking what feels like 'right action' in the direction of positive change and wholeness offers a way to be a part of a solution.

Similar to identifying which part of your system is most responsible for the symptom, it's helpful to find the doors in the community that are most likely to be open to the change that needs to happen. It might be a person, an office, or organization who possibly is already set up to get things in motion in a new direction. Old ways of doing things, just like old ways of being, can create discomfort during transitions. When your posture has been off for a few years, the correct posture will feel odd initially, until the proprioceptors adapt to the change. The compensatory patterns made the imbalance feel normal, but when you look in the mirror, you can see that it's actually off. In a few days, however, the new balance takes pressure off your spine, hips, and other joints and feels amazing.

Social stressors and pressures are a leading cause of many types of illness, but there's no need to feel that they must all be corrected in society first for you to come to balance and heal. In fact, Native American elders generally say to heal yourself first. Somatic blindness can lead to the 'imagined' type of pressure; the self-inflicted type that exists as an internal habit, no longer in the presence of a real threat. This type is often accompanied by other layers of unconsciousness in the psyche that makes it challenging to turn on the light to see oneself. When deadlines are present, workloads are high, a headache is raging, co-workers are flipping out, and there's little time left to sort out your thoughts and feelings; there's another layer of pressure that can build from personal issues not being resolved.

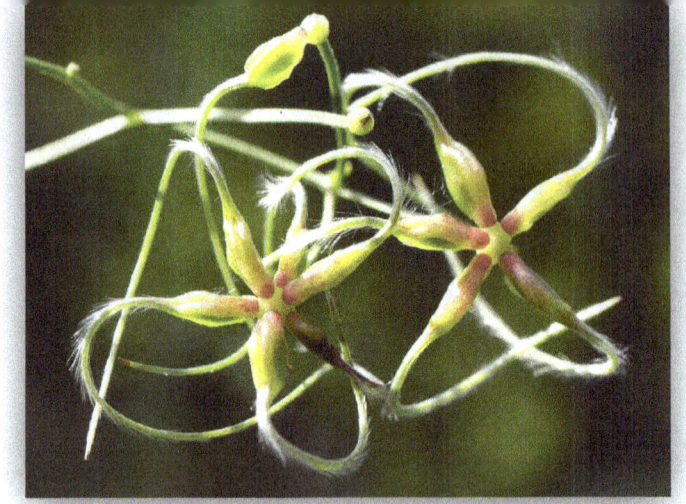

Social pressure is more difficult to discern because it's imbedded and situational with many moving parts. There may be an outer object or person to blame it on - particularly with institutionalized 'isms,' but it may not relieve the pressure because the person or 'ism' isn't the same as the wound. Naming the cause seems relieving for the mind, but not if it isn't true. You may think someone is judging you for the zit on your face, or because you're a woman, but it may not be true. We are often our own worst critic. The tendency may be to project, but it's more empowering to accept responsibility for your reaction as an impartial witness to your reaction. That can change how your mind reacts. Taking a moment to check in and promise to look at how the pressure is living inside your body is a huge benefit. Making an appointment with a manual therapist to help unpack it is often very relieving. You can discover movements that can help unwind internalized pressures and change how your body reacts. Now the stress is reduced and personal solutions can be uncovered. The answers were always similar: take care of the body, become more aware and compassionate, and form a clear plan of action that feels balanced.

For my pressured situations at work, whether the issue was tackling repairs, with personality disputes, staffing shortages and trainings, administrative backlogs, client satisfaction, financial issues, flash flood warnings, co-worker illnesses, and deaths, the answers were never built in. There was always a learning curve that was challenging to feel at the top of. Yet the answer in such a wide variety of situations always came down to my willingness to be more present and let the information for each unique issue sink in, and have the patience for the solution to show itself. A growing acceptance of surfing a wave that was never the same helped tremendously, along with realizing that the water was moving in a certain direction already. A lot of the pressure came from trying to swim upstream with ideas that weren't being supported yet by current circumstances.

Even if the pressure was from old classics like relationships, discrimination, or finances, the solutions were not always cut and dry, particularly if you couldn't see an easy exit. It also helped to see that my brain could just feed forward a list of

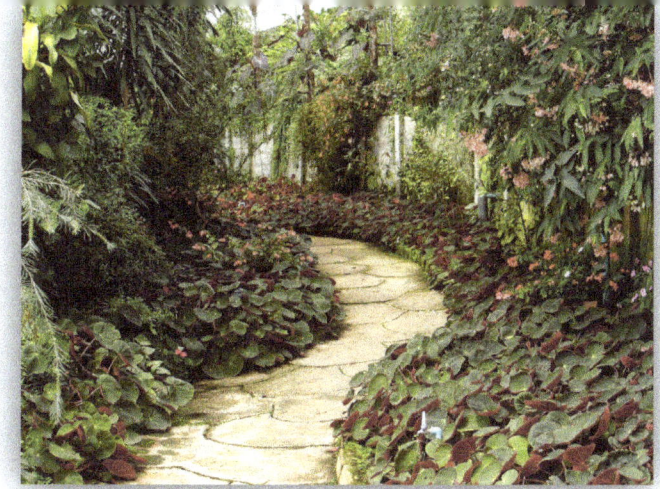

pros and cons that didn't in themselves amount to the right decision on how to handle it. That slogan to 'sleep on it' made more and more sense, as input from the subtle bodies would make their way down into my conscious mind during the night and the solutions would be there in the morning. I just had to be present and listen for the download as it trickled in through the quiet. The right decision usually included something that felt like the right thing to do, and followed right timing. Using this as a guiding principle kept me aligned with my body, heart, and energy, which was more wholesome and healthier internally. It didn't always sit well with everyone involved, but the best answer wasn't always the one that made everyone happy. It had to feel right for the whole, and make sense considering whatever resources were currently available. What seemed like the wisest approach to take had to prove itself to be true in action, or be reevaluated down the road if it didn't.

**Self-talk,** (a potential form of imagined pressure) then changed into a conversation that supported organization towards a goal, and the understanding that I'd learn how to get there along the way, which had a little pressure built in. In that sense I'd always felt unprepared, but had clear goals. It was challenging to get my body and intellect functioning well again, but once the subconscious stumbling blocks were reorganized, life began to flow. I could get a sense of where the pressures were creating contractions in my system, and develop movements to unwind them before joint restrictions or compressions became a nuisance. You can say that your body will open more when your mind does, but it's even more true that your mind will open more when your body does. Both open with consciousness.

I learned to hold my thoughts blameless because they appeared to be reflections of how my body was feeling, even when they were reacting to thoughts coming towards me. My body was registering the pressure, using thoughts as a language to echo the tension. Consciousness is always already free and exists unfettered as awareness in the background of every experience. Consciousness doesn't have an opinion, but has ever-shining, clear eyes to see with. I was gradually learning to sit back in that quality of consciousness and receive fresh insights from there. From there the personality is also full of files to draw from, but is also a fluid medium

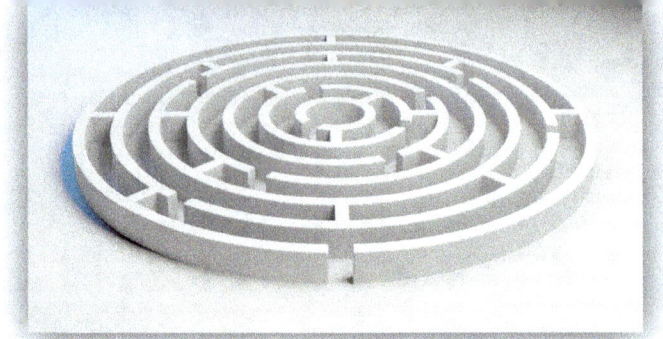

through which to express healthier decisions that are not laced with history. From that point on, for the last 35 years, there hasn't been a recurrence of depression or lingering emotional states. It's then just a matter of being present day-to-day to discharge stressors, optimize perception, and surf the waves of experiencing.

## Discerning types of pain

After I felt more human as a being, I could dial into healing this basket full of injuries. Figuring out pain types admittedly took some time and practice, trial and error, a ton of concentration, and contemplation with detachment. The detachment part that developed, or was gifted by Grace, enabled many of the revelations and insights to happen the way that they did. It's almost impossible to see clearly while leaning all the way into pain. We all have that Grace within, even if you don't have an external Spiritual figure in your life. In addition, I was supremely motivated and eternally curious and fascinated by what was being revealed. Listening to your body's intelligence with an intent to learn transforms the experience, and opens a new wave of inspiration to explore further. There are zillions of pathways and types of communication happening all the time in our systems, some bearing sensations that are different from those we're used to experiencing.

There aren't words for them in our vocabulary, but they do have a sensation that can be remembered, associated in context, and learned from. One of the factors that was revelatory during a type of pain that became depression 40 years ago, was to objectify it as a state and tune into to see where it was in my body and feel into it. It felt like nothing, and I was used to feeling something. It was super quiet, like a void or vacuum, and there were no thoughts in it telling me that my life sucked, or that I sucked, or that my situation sucked—nothing; just dead silence. I began to think, "This is actually a lovely little quiet cave that I can rest inside of. Maybe what I need is rest. Maybe my system just crashed because I've been physically and emotionally overloaded for a long time and I should respect that".

When I took a step back and looked objectively at the situations that led up to the state and felt into the state itself, I felt compassion for my body. It had really withstood a lot with reduced resources to do so and it was understandable that it wanted to shut itself down for a bit. I let myself lie in the quiet of it for a while - can't

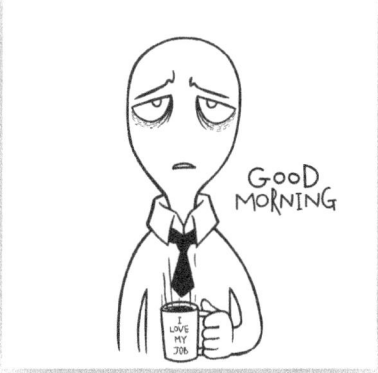

remember if it was hours, days, or weeks - then faced into the driving forces behind the crash. I remembered a woman who said she was psychic telling me, "You need to eat!" I also remembered a nurse telling me at the hospital when I checked myself into an emergency room after fainting and hitting my head, "Your blood pressure is so low it's amazing you're still alive!" I think my blood pressure was something like 70/50 instead of 90/60 like it usually was.

Those brief statements re-entered my consciousness as if my body was trying to send me another malnutrition message. This time it was much clearer. Pain, weakness, depression, negative thoughts and irritability didn't get the message across, but hearing those words again inside my head did. These were the early stages of becoming interested in creating a better relationship with my body and learning to listen in a new way. Change in mood, change of sleep patterns, or thought patterns are all messages from the body. The next step after receiving the message would be to pause and ask, "What do you need?"

There were times when rest was really the answer, and I'd been the type to burn candles at both ends as well as the middle simultaneously for decades. I knew the energy was there, but it took a while to distinguish physical vitality from energy. I had learned to draw from a Universal life force that was always available, but it still was not a good idea to run my body into the ground. It was sort of like using an external generator when the power is out, but the generator is covering up the fact that the power is out. I think we all have a reserve tank, but it's not healthy to empty that one on a regular basis. Survival needs kept the engine running for a while, but days off were about nothing but rest. The body didn't have juice for anything else.

**Fatigue** can present as a form of pain. Pain as blocked energy can make you feel drained, and stress can do the same. When clients presented with chronic fatigue as an illness, there was usually an emotional component that was unresolved. Withdrawal, retreat, and freeze are all part of the hypo side of the nervous system. We're used to seeing the hyper side of things with stress, but the other gets less press. If you can identify the felt sense of perceived fatigue in your body, the source of it will identify itself, come to the surface, and begin the release.

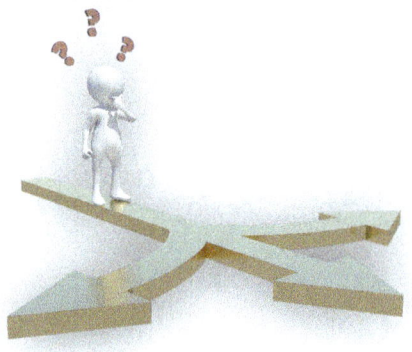

As time went on and discernment increased, I could sift through the zillions of bits of information being processed to dial in more specifically which system was fatigued. It's sort of like being on a busy street and locating which car was honking its horn. That's how I was able to tell which type of breakfast dropped my energy, or that my eyes were fatigued, my heart was overloaded, my back needed rest or massage, or that my feet were compressed. The heart, according to recent studies in neurophysics, stores the largest amount of memory. I was astonished how much stuff released while I contemplated the field. As the energy dissipated, so did little aches and pains elsewhere. Sometimes when one part needs attention it will feel like the entire body is drained, but it isn't. I felt normal energy everywhere else in these instances, and learned how to address the part and restore it to the whole.

Pain can be a tremendous pressure cooker and barrier to being able to make conscious decisions. I've met clients who've endured tremendous amounts of pain for many years, without being able to track down the cause. Luckily, they'd kept trying. Pain can either function as a motivator to act, or become a paralyzing event. Therefore, it helps to be able to distinguish and discern different types of pain as a way of knowing which action to take. There are many instances when there will be no precipitating event that you can identify, yet some pain is there with a new type of sensation that you don't recognize. I'm hoping that my experiences can help save some time for others in figuring out the different types, with the understanding that each system has a different history, so you'll know that a similar situation might send a different signal in your system.

You can use these examples as a loose frame of reference. Stress started early in my life. As a teenager, a sharp pain developed in my chest and went up through my neck on the left side. It was a little scary so my mother took me to the doctor. Turns out it was gas. I'd have never imagined that gas would produce sensations that high up in the body, but the medication he gave me for gas worked. I also learned then that the stress producing gastro-intestinal distress, could make you think you're having a heart attack. It could also produce rashes, which I'd developed around the same time.

It's helpful for parents to be aware of these signals when they arise, so deeper probing can happen. Children may not know what to do about it. Nonetheless, the

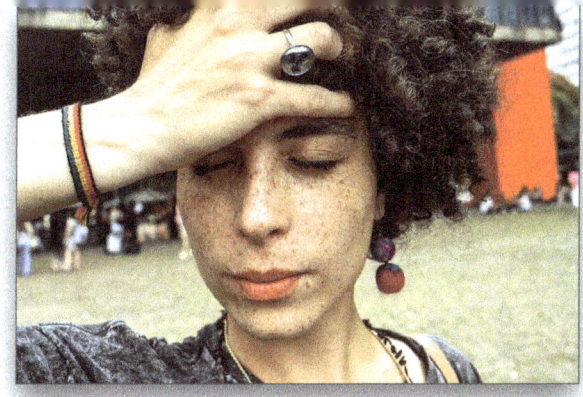

association of that sensation with gas stayed with me, and was useful as a frame of reference when it happened again later in life. I'm often surprised at the amount of tension and contraction children in elementary school have in their bodies. When they speak about all of the activities they're involved in, particularly those dancing ballet, doing gymnastics, or playing sports, it's not so surprising. Adults often are under the assumption that young bodies shouldn't be experiencing stress or tension and don't do anything to help them feel better. The type of soreness that arises out of muscle tissue being torn down and rebuilt doesn't have age limits.

There's much less soreness after working out when there's more oxygen available, and it will be even less if your system isn't tight to begin with. **Ischemia**, or lack of oxygen in the tissue, happens when tight muscles or bound up fascia restrict blood flow. At times massage can resolve the issue, but other times, myofascial work may be more appropriate. If it's a pattern, like in thoracic outlet syndrome, it's best to have the restriction removed specifically around the arteries in question, as well as in the related soft tissue fields. It can also happen that neighboring bones have become slightly displaced and are generating soft tissue tension. Sensations of numbness down the arm into the hand could be a nerve supply issue from the brachial plexus at the base of the neck, but it could also be caused by a vascular restriction. It's best to explore different options as to the source of the restriction.

**Numbness** and loss of sensation are distinguishable from sciatica, for example, where a nerve is pinched and is radiating pain down part or all of the nerve into the foot. In either case, when there are nerve signs of numbness, tingling, pinching, or radiating pain, it's best to see someone to take care of the restriction rather than use a painkiller alone. There are different types of pain medication as well, and some are better suited to nerve pain than others. Continuing to do daily life tasks while on painkillers runs the risk of further injuring the area in question. I often used hypericum, ginger or Serrapeptase for nerve pain to help reduce inflammation.

**Irritated trigger points** - usually where a nerve enters a muscle - can also send radiating pain that can be searing, sharp, or tender. These can throw you off because the origin of the trigger point may not be near the referred area where you feel it the most. There are trigger point maps out there you can look at in order to help figure out if it relates to your situation, and you can even try to treat it by

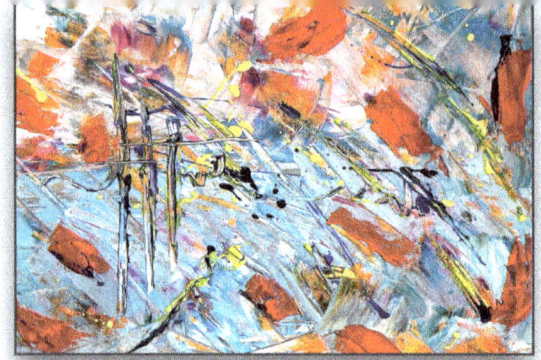

applying gentle pressure to the point a few times to see if the pain decreases. If not, it's best to see someone sooner rather than later so that an inflammatory pattern doesn't progress into something worse.

**Headaches** are very common and can have a variety of causes. Vascular issues, as previously mentioned, are a fairly common cause of pain and tension, as can be the case for headaches. Discerning which soft or bony tissue is responsible for the reduced blood flow will be useful. Reduced flow in or out of the brain can produce pressure, as can restrictions in movement of the cranial bones, or tension or torsions in membranes around or within the brain. These same types of restrictions may cause neck tension that can further exert pressures on the skull resulting in a headache. A lesser known contributor is the jaw muscles that tie into the temporalis muscle in the face, and the membranes that exert forces on the skull.

Clenching or grinding teeth at night are often unsuspecting sources of tension that can build into a headache. Since headaches are so common, people very often don't seek help other than a Tylenol or Ibuprofen. Pain and inflammation can be connected since inflammation is the body's first responder when there's an issue. One such client who'd been on 10 Tylenol a day for 10 years went down to 2 a day after working with her, but high doses of niacin (suggested by a medical intuitive) set her free. She'd tried many things over the years. That last percentage was an internal issue that needed nutritional support with the ability to open the vasculature from within. People do have chronic headaches, such as cluster headaches, but only because they haven't uncovered the cause. I've seen them resolve with proper motion of the parietal bones on the side of the skull, but there may be other causes as well.

For **tension headaches**, which many will experience at work, a good question to ask is, "Where is the tension that's pulling on my neck, or skull, or dura (underneath the skull) to create the headache?" It can be as far away as your feet, or hips, or as near as the suboccipital muscles. These are the clarifications that will reveal themselves once you begin to hone self-sensing skills within the conversations you'll be having with your system. There are a few common places to look that are usually responsible, but it's way better to know how your system in

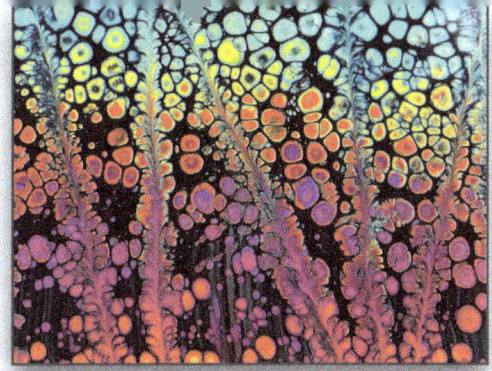

particular functions. You can definitely test out the others in the beginning, just to rule them in or out if you're not trusting your discernment sensibilities yet.

The main areas to look in general initially are fascial chains. There's a posterior chain that runs from the feet up the back of the legs and hamstrings, up the sacrum, spine and neck all the way to the head. Tension along any part of the chain could pull the rest of the way up, but if you're sitting long hours, you can start with the hamstrings. If you spend long hours on your feet, check the lateral chain that runs up the side of the legs through the IT band, across the hips and up the spine to the head. If the IT band isn't letting go, you will want to open the lateral knee joint and possibly the peroneus muscles in the lower leg first, particularly if you have high arches. Another key area that affects many people is the upper traps because they originate at the base of the skull.

People who spend long hours at a computer will often have complaints of tension there, or in the **eyes** which are reflexive with the suboccipital muscles, which can easily pull on the skull and even tweak internal membranes. In realizing that the brain, skull, and attaching connective tissue are real anatomical structures that are part of a larger fabric of tissue fields, you might feel curious to sense where your main corresponding tightness is and open it back up before the headache sets in, even if it's from stress. The wonderful part about attuning to the body's language is that you do get early warnings in a variety of ways. One test you can use for yourself is to stick your tongue out and see if it pulls more to one side or not. The back of the tongue could let you know which side of the deeper connective tissue in your throat may be a source of tension that could exert forces on and around dural membranes beneath the skull through to the upper cervical region. Gargling might help to loosen some of these areas effectively and easy enough to experiment with. You can also just stretch your tongue in all directions and see what that does, both to reveal tension sources, and possibly alleviate them.

**Migraines** and hormonal headaches are related to a different system. Some women experience migraines around the time of the menses and are usually incapacitated by them. Some believe that the liver is implicated in migraines, and because the liver is involved in the regulation of hormones, it does make sense that this would be a good spot to look. It's not a bad idea to do a liver cleanse from

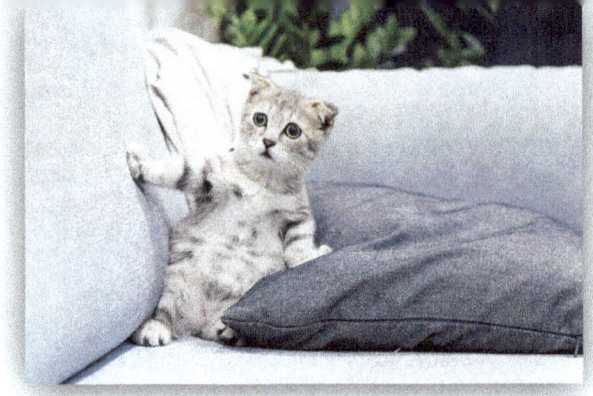

time to time, or take a liver tonic, and check your diet and meds for which might be toxic for the liver. There are also foods that support liver function. When I had a hemiplegic (one-sided) migraine after a concussion, it was mostly due to the irritation of cranial nerves and inflammation that had gotten set forth from the brain injury and tissue damage. Nerve pain can be excruciating and nearly intolerable at times. The eyes are often a good place to have someone check for help with migraines, along with the associated nuclei in the brain.

**Inflammation** is natural when an injury is in the healing process, and is best treated with ice, as there is already additional heat from biochemical processes. While in that tender phase, it's often best to rest the injury. This was an invaluable 'study' in becoming able to distinguish the different types of pain and then know which ones I could stretch or apply pressure to, or approach indirectly, take anti-inflammatories for, use essential oils for, or best served with cardiovascular exercise. The body might feel fatigued when inflammation is present, in order to weaken you so you won't be inclined to overdo it while it's trying to mend itself. The other benefits that come with recovering from injury to the central nervous system are that you are able to more deeply appreciate the miracle that is the incredible fragility, suppleness, intelligence, and paradoxical strength of the system.

**Nausea** can accompany a brain injury or migraine as the vagus nerve where it sits in the carotid sheath can become irritated and be felt in the belly. Although you can take something to ease the nausea, it's better to release the pressure on the vagus nerve. I found that using very gentle myofascial work on the carotid sheath in the neck, while feeling into that tight, burning sensation coming from the nerve until it settles and opens, offers a more permanent resolution. Ginger and peppermint have been known to help with nausea as well as with headaches. Gentle, global movement that opens the cervical muscles is also helpful.

**Dull, deep aches** can cause clients to complain and become concerned when it's in or around a joint. A tear in the joint capsule might create a deep ache, but if there's a point where you can't move it any further, there might be a tear inside. Steroid injections can help for a while, and some manage without surgery. **Bursitis** can also create a deep ache in a joint, and some say that type of inflammation responds well to yucca extract. I had it in my hip joint and yucca did a great job.

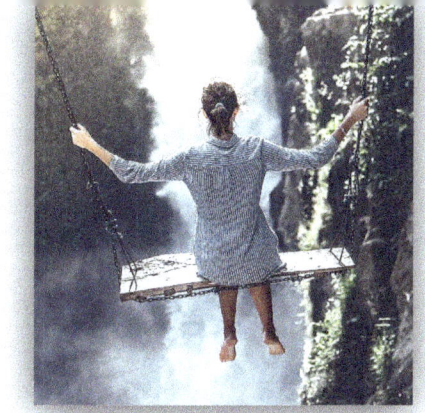

Cramps from menses may bring the sensation of a dull ache across the low back and belly as well. Consider checking the lumbar vertebrae for compression as those nerves feed forward into the pelvic bowl. Pressure from fluid build-up or restricted movement can be part of the pain, and opening the space around the uterus and in the lower abdomen in general can help alleviate these symptoms. Moist heat can help deep aches. Infrared light may also be beneficial.

**Frozen shoulder, or adhesive capsulitis,** has many different types of pain associated with it, because so many muscles in the area contract. The surest way to determine if that's what's going on is to check your range of motion. If you can lift your arm over your head and put it behind your back, it's not frozen. If you can only lift it part way, particularly if you've had a stressful event or are in menopause, you can turn it around with treatment. If it locks all the way it could take a while to self-correct even with treatment, but you can move through the process without much pain. It tends to get worse if you reach away from your body quickly. A sharp pain usually follows right behind that action. If you reach slowly every time, and carefully and don't try to go out beyond 30-45 degrees, you'll likely experience very little discomfort as you regain your range of motion.

**Kidneys** can produce a dull ache when they feel overloaded, or when they are being compressed by the psoas and quadratus lumborum muscles in the back. It's easy to mistake this for a backache, but it might be remedied by mobilizing the kidney. Until you've discovered the source of the dull, deep ache it's best not to over-exert yourself in case something is on an edge of becoming damaged. As you become more and more familiar with the types of pain your body expresses in a variety of circumstances, you'll know what's safe to do or not, and eliminate the guesswork. Ultrasound could rule out whether it's a kidney issue.

**Sharp, stinging types of gripping pain** can come from fascial adhesions as the layers are attempting to peel apart, but can't without help. It's best to go slowly after the initial contact with the sting, allowing the body to recognize the restriction and unwind it on its own terms. Forcing the issue might create a tear, which will then take a while to repair. The same applies to stretching, as you don't want to force the issue is the body expresses a barrier with this type of restriction. Another possibility is that the tissue is reacting to an energetic blockage. These areas can also produce a sharp, stinging sensation. Try opening entry and exit points for meridians, or connect two similar spots with the pulsing method and see if it changes things. Check with a professional beforehand if you're in doubt.

**Emotional** pain can become tied in to physical pain, and can sometimes be the cause of it. Emotional pain is more draining than physical pain and is more resistant to analgesics, but responds well to movement and exercise. It will often sit in the upper chest or create heaviness in the belly and brain. You can also check the heart and lung meridians. Emotional pain after grief after a loss can be episodic as the memories connected with things you shared become unhinged and rise to be released. There are many beautiful ways to celebrate these memories, and to embrace the release of where they sit in your cells. It is a gorgeous process to let this type of sadness wash through your system on its way out.

Some of my clients have been in stages of decision-making for quite a while, while others are ready to decide right away. There are times when the conscious mind seems ready, but the emotional or unconscious layer isn't ready yet. As you begin to sense into the different types of sensations and tensions and move into them, those experiences may reveal a face or a voice of the past. Choice points will arise again and again as you have a fresh chance to make a decision on what you want to keep, what you want to modify, and what you want to release. Understanding how information becomes stored in the unconscious or subconscious parts of ourselves can be a significant factor in you being able to make a clearer, healthier decision.

# Chapter 4

## Establishing a Baseline

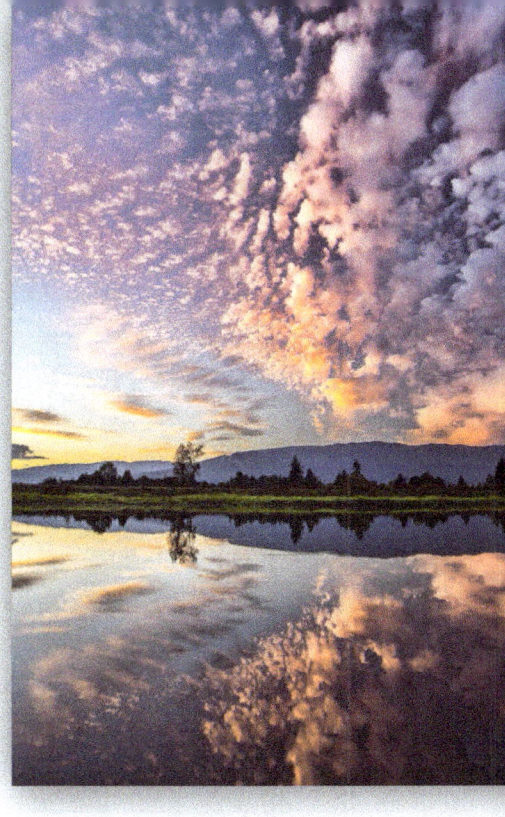

Our bodies function as a whole, in an intimate relationship with all of its parts. I want to encourage you to learn your body's language so you can discover what wholeness feels like. Feeling whole is deeper and fuller than being comfortable in your body. It includes the spectrum between the thickest, most dense parts of us, to the finest, most subtle spaces that bring you significant information about your energetic well-being. Building a deeper connection with your system is going to be a tremendous help in turning around or preventing health issues from developing, but will also align you with your Spirit.

In order to support this level of well-being on a regular basis, you'll need to establish a baseline resting tone so that you know what 'normal' feels like. Even if, and especially if you've been healthy, you probably don't pay attention to what that state feels like. There may not be an adjective for what balanced anatomy feels like, but you can still sense it. Our systems make a 'noise' when they're out of balance, but just have a little 'hum' when all is well. It's like being in a quiet room with a lamp plugged in instead of a fridge. It may be even more like being outside in a garden on a warm day, or out on a lake in a small boat. It feels calmly vital and rich, plush and peaceful with many forms of life that are in sync.

That said, let's go through a practice of discovering for yourself what it's like for you. If you do feel some little aches or pains, we'll use the language of contrasting sensations as a way to guide your system into a more neutral space. What happens along with the sensing, will be your awareness waking up your brain as to what's happening. If you have never tuned into your body and feel at a loss for how to be in touch with its sensors, make a fist and feel the sensation of your knuckles, fingers, palms, and fingernails. Squeeze your thighs and see how deeply into your leg you're able to sense, and notice what the internal sensation feels like.

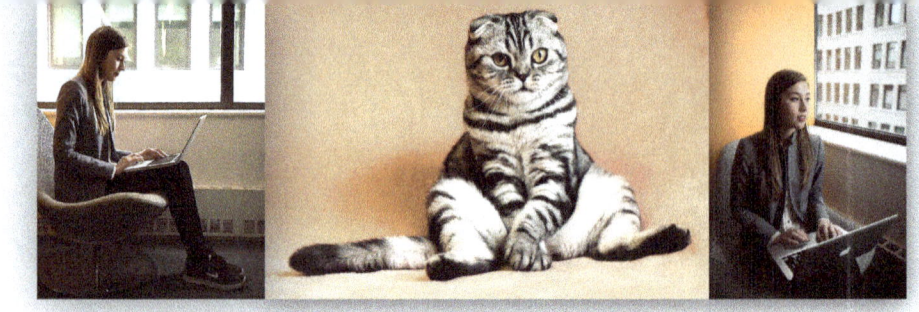

## Getting a sense of things while sitting

First, find a comfortable chair to sit in that's not too firm, but also not so cushy that your hips will be uneven. If you're completely new at self-sensing and haven't tuned in to tactile kinesthetic sensations at all, you can check out the exercises in volume 4 of this series, or follow along this sequence and know that like with any new activity, it gets better and easier with practice and repetition. Start by getting a sense of what it is that you're sitting on, and let a few adjectives float through your consciousness to describe that surface. Is it flexible or stiff, cool or room temperature? Is the surface smooth or if there is a texture to the surface that you can detect, how would you describe it? Ribbed, velour, satiny, leathery, pile, woven, and does it feel thick or thin? Is there something beneath the upholstery that you can sense into and make note of a few of its qualities?

Is it holding you easily upright or is it form-fitting? Is what you're wearing agreeing with the surface you're sitting on; are there any wrinkles or uneven areas in your skirt, dress, or pants that may make the surfaces work against one another? If so, take a moment to straighten them out so that there is barely, if any, noticeable difference between them. Make note of your skin against the fabric you have on and any adjectives you can use to describe how it feels to you, or how your skin feels in direct contact with the chair if that's the case. If there's an imbalance in how the tissue is lying on the chair so that there's a pull more in one direction than another, adjust your legs and hips so that both thighs feel more evenly balanced on the chair.

Notice how the 'sit' bones or ischial tuberosities feel on the surface of the seat. Is one side bearing more weight than the other? If so, shift them until they feel equal in weight bearing. Is one side sore or experiencing more sensation than the other? If so, is that a new sensation, or the first time you're noticing it? Are your knees level with the surface of the chair, or are they a little or lower than the edge of the chair? If the pressure on the hamstrings in the back of your thighs is in any way uncomfortable, adjust with more or fewer pillows until it feels good. Adjust the position of your feet so that the toes are square, or point them inward or outward slightly while checking the response in your knees and hips. Are your feet altogether comfortable in your shoes if you're wearing any?

Are there any pressure places of the shoes on your toes or anywhere else that can be made more comfortable? If you're wearing socks, are they absolutely smooth inside the shoe? Find an adjective or two to describe the texture of your socks or skin against the shoes or the floor, whichever is the case for you. Find a way to sink into the shoes and feel through them into the floor so that there's a seamless meeting and harmony between all of these layers. We're waking up the mechanoreceptors (sensors) in your body while also waking up your awareness in these areas. You will discover how they feel in and of themselves, as well as in relationship to their immediate surroundings.

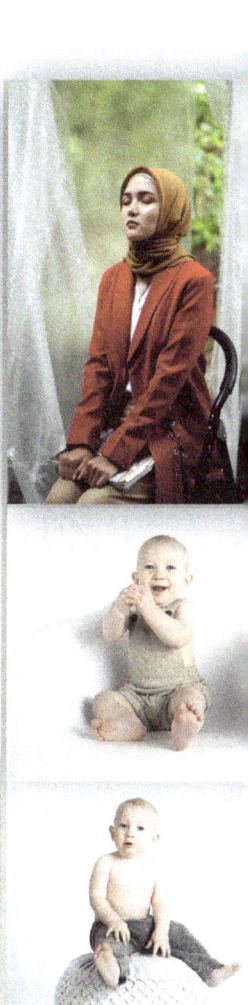

This is enabling your brain and you to re-evaluate what's happening and to reeducate the tense places. The closer attention you pay to each area, the more it will reveal to you. Making small, mindful movements will also expose relationships that have played a role in the tension you've been experiencing. You may find that some areas are working harder than others. The areas working the hardest will usually be the most sore. The first relationship we'll sense is the one between your feet, your knees, and the floor. Do a brief scan initially to see if any one area stands out above another. It may be your heels, a particular toe or instep; it could be the knee cap, or shin bone between the foot and the knee.

Once you've found a tight spot, for example, in your knee, make little adjustments in your feet until that area becomes a neutral place with minimal or no sensation. Rotate your feet internally and externally just a hair while monitoring slight changes in comfort in the ankles, up the legs, and into the joints. Adjust your feet until you feel complete comfort between the soles of your feet and the floor. Check the points of contact and see if anything can be improved. Lift your feet so your toes are closer to the shin bone. Do you feel some tightness in your calf muscles?

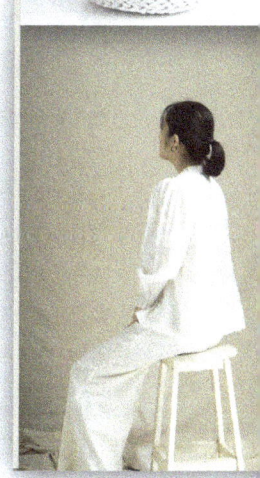

Is there more tension on the surface, or in deeper layers of the calf muscle? Squeeze the muscle if you can't feel the interior of it yet. Next, lift your heels until you're on the balls of your feet and sense the (anterior tibialis) muscle next to the shin bone. Notice if it pulls through its tendon down into the instep. Do this motion three times as slowly as you can, lifting onto the balls of the feet, then rocking back onto your heels and lifting the feet towards the shins. Visualize your feet passing through a huge body of water that opens into a puffy cloud in the sky that has the magical ability of infusing its light, airy qualities in between the bones.

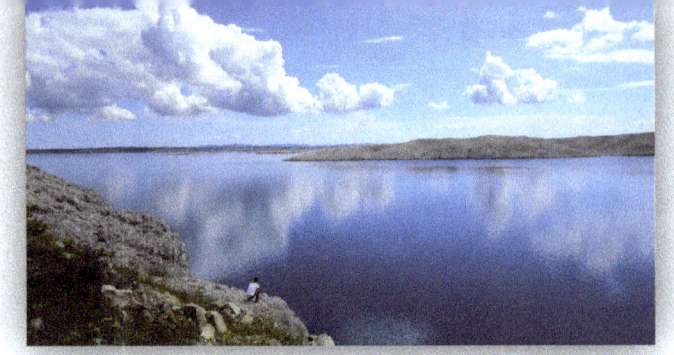

Check in again after this visualization and note if there are any remaining areas that stick out from the rest. We're aiming for calm neutral from the surface, through the feet up into the knees. If there are sensations, try to become specific in what type of sensation it is; find an adjective if you can. Does it feel sharp, dull, burning, itchy, scratchy, irritable, tense, thick, knotted, bound up, stiff, or wound up? Isolate the location as much as you can while maintaining your attention on the entire foot and leg. Then, as gently and gradually as you can, internally and externally rotate the lower leg, and roll your foot over onto the outer edge, then inner arch, and notice what happens for the entire lower leg.

As you move, go back and forth, and side-to-side until you discover the position of the most ease for the foot and leg and stay there. As you make these tiny adjustments in search of the most balanced status, your body will echo your intention and begin release compensatory patterns in the leg that you may not have been aware of. Allow a couple of minutes to track those internal corrections. When you and your system are really in sync, if you initiate a tiny motion towards the tension your body will complete the inquiry for you with its own self-regulatory mechanisms. The body is always self-sensing, but can only make so many adjustments once it's become laden with years of patterns that have become counter-productive. Your body is learning to tune in to the minutia in your tissue fields at the same time that you are.

Remember that you are waking those areas up out of numbing sensory-motor amnesia, after which your brain will redistribute the workload of the muscles and connective tissue accordingly. Once awakened, the area will be able to send more accurate information to itself about what's happening from moment-to-moment. You may find that there is a slight delay between when the information you are sending (by slightly altering your position) reaches the brain, to the time when the body receives that input and sends down its own adjustments. Wait for the changes to feedforward from the brain. Continue after you feel the changes.

Really let the image of the watery sky with clouds become infused into your joints. Spend a moment at each place until you feel the joint accept the image by the felt-sense of a shift inside of it. Allow the image to spill over into your bones and soft tissue, with the blueness of the sky representing oxygen flow throughout your

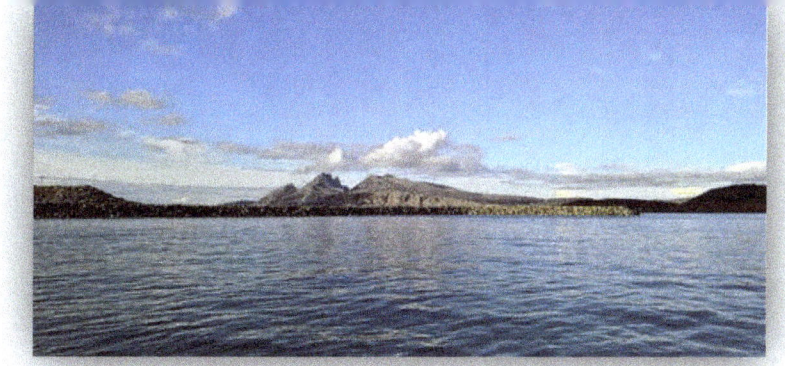

muscles and connective tissue. I used this image of the blueness being oxygen once when recovering from the disc injury while spending time on the StairMaster and it made a huge difference right away. A new burst of energy came into my entire system from using that visualization, making me feel like the frequency of the color blue meant something to the body in its own language.

Now that the relationships in the lower body have been recalibrated, follow the sensations you notice up your thighs and into the hip joints and pelvis. Find the most neutral position for the areas in the entire lower body as they relate to the chair you're sitting on. When there's a perfect balance it should begin to feel like the seat and floor are comfy appendages to your hips, legs, and feet. Sway a tiny bit forward and back pivoting on the hip joints keeping your back straight. Seek and find a spot for your spine over your pelvis and sacrum that feels ideal for balance.

See if there's a spot that makes sitting upright feel effortless and pick the one that comes the closest. We do have effortless posture when we're much younger, and if we feel into and release those unnecessary forces creating tension, that easeful posture can return. An enormous amount of energy is continually being used to renegotiate poor posture all over the system, and particularly in the spine. Tension in the spine is often connected to uneven pulls created by the shoes we wear, so it's wise to reorganize peripheral areas first, then see what's left in the core - our midline. Energetic and mechanical forces sent from your hands and feet into the spine can be substantial. Every move you make with them will affect the core. Try opening your hands to the sky and earth with arms and legs outstretched to empty excess energy before beginning this exercise. You might be pleasantly surprised.

## Negotiating torsion

Art imitates life in many instances, as the structures expressed by living beings are by their nature functionally practical and sound. Tissue fields develop in spirals, at times in accordance with the dimensions of phi, also known as the Golden Ratio. That said, there are times when our gait, the way our shoes are shaped inside, the shape of our bones in the lower legs, or even the pull of the hip flexing psoas muscle attaching on the femur will generate a slight twist in the pelvis. If there is a

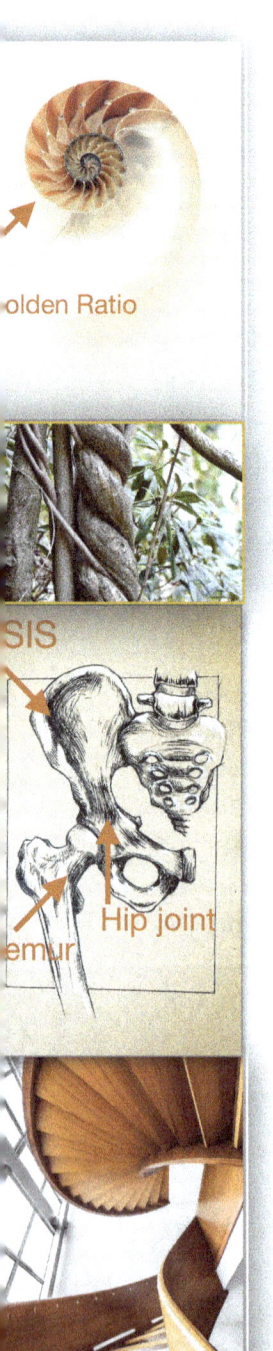

twist in the pelvis, it means that the shoulder, neck and head will counter-rotate to re-establish balance. As discussed earlier, a rotation on the spine as well as within any joint, increases the pounds of pressure on the disc immensely, so try not to leave that rotation in your body.

One way to check is if you feel an increased tension in the quad or hamstring on one side. A tight quad could rotate the ilium down in the front, while a tight hamstring could pull it down on one side in the back. Anatomical markers can reveal a rotation if you place your fingers on the ASIS (anterior superior iliac spine) on each side and compare where they are. If one is higher than the other, it's rotated. If one side is farther forward than the other, you also have a rotated pelvis. It's not uncommon for there to be a rotation in two directions at the same time. Because it's so common I speculate that it's from driving, but that's just speculation; a number of things could cause it.

may also depend upon which types of compensatory patterns and restrictions are already in place as to who may or may not develop these spirals. As a test, let's take a moment now that you have a resting baseline and can more easily sense a change in status. Tune in to your lower body again, sensing into your legs, hip joints, and pelvis. Pretend you're driving so that the lower leg will be slightly extended towards where the pedal would be. From here, dorsiflex (lift) your right foot towards the shin like you'd do if you were about to step on the gas. Check the effects in the hip, then check again while lifting the entire foot before you put it down. Repeat the same on the other side and make note of the differences between sides. Be sure the surface you're sitting on isn't tilting your pelvis and distorting the results. In many cars the seats tilt the pelvis, producing issues in the hips or sacroiliac joints as a consequence.

This was true in my car, and using a cushion did the same thing in a different way. If you drive for long periods or carry your wallet in your back pocket, over time you might notice some stiffness and soreness develop in the low back. After repeating this exercise a few times, could you tell how your pelvic bones were changing position? I noticed that it felt like my right side was relaxing with each effort, while the left side added a little more tension each time. Each time the left side delivered more feedback about the position of the iliac crest than the right side, which like it was buried under a layer of sand. After repeating the movement a few times, the right side offered more sensation; it felt more awake and aware.

Take inventory of how your body responded and apply those observations the next time you're in your car, seated at a restaurant, or watching a movie. Whatever the situation is, it makes a tremendous difference if you stay in touch with what's going on in your body. At least tune in from time to time, so that you can make little adjustments along the way. Otherwise, you could feel like it's not as easy as it used to be changing from sitting to standing, and blame the creakiness on age.

Whether you're playing the piano, designing a floor plan, or whatever might put you in this position, practice getting in and out of the seat as smoothly as you can. Play with a few positions until you find the most balanced posture for you. Workstation ergonomics has become a big deal in recent years due to the amount of injuries that were occurring. Some are caused by reaching for something, like a phone or calculator, by rotating the upper body towards it while the lower body stays in the same position. If that happens to be your situation, consider swiveling the entire chair to face whatever it is you need so that you're not twisting at the waist. Remember that your intestines are being torqued as well. Check for rebalance options during your time being seated, or if not then, do so at the end of your shift so that the forces created can be released.

According to some folks who study the ergonomics of the seated position, the position of the legs in relation to the pelvis when on a horse is supposed to be ideal. The spine rests easily atop the sacrum when the thighs are at the 60 rather than a 90-degree angle to the pelvis. There are saddle chairs out there these days that, if the cushion is just right, is ergonomically correct and very comfortable for a while. It's best to get up and move around as soon as you feel fatigue. For most people in Western culture, the back will fatigue after a couple of hours without the option to lean back once in a while. Also, in a saddle chair it would be more difficult for the torsion to occur because there's something between your legs. It's smaller, and the constant movement underneath you will provoke continual adaptation by your upper body, which is a good thing. Torsions can be corrected for you by a manual therapist, or you can also familiarize yourself with the landmarks and move in ways that correct it for yourself.

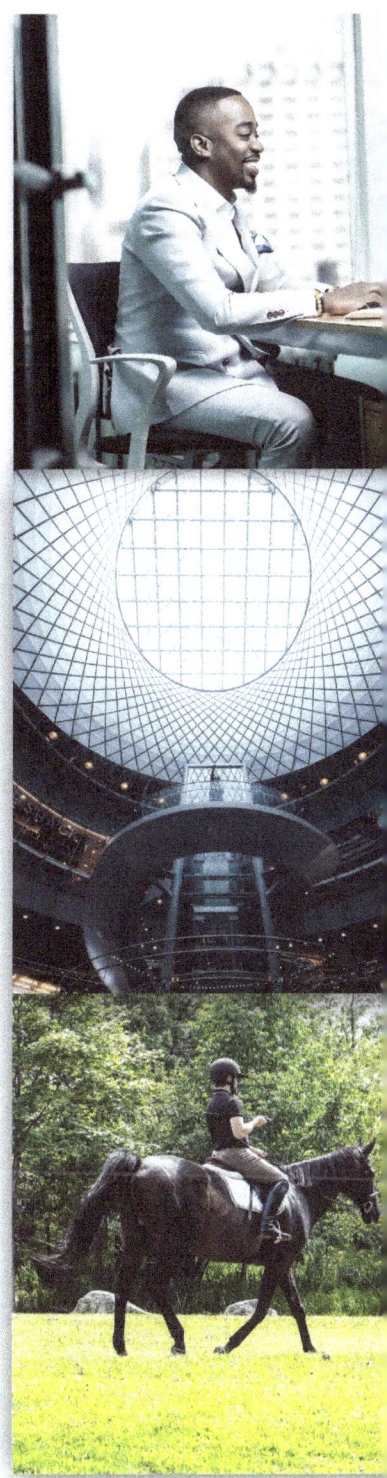

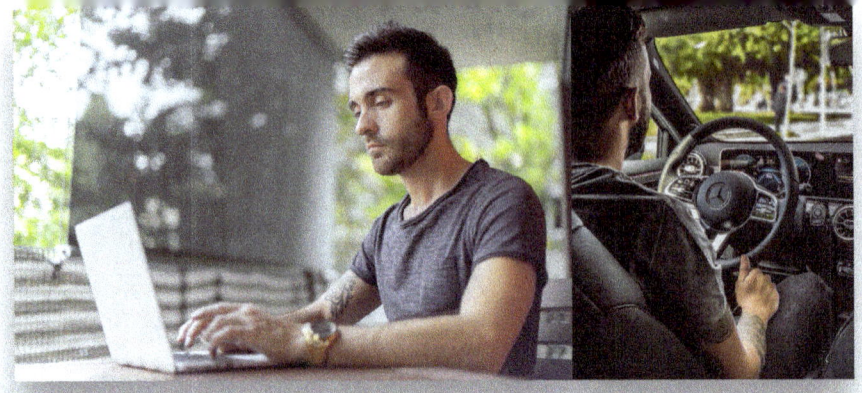

While being seated now, notice each side of the ASIS at the most forward tip of the iliac crest, then slide each knee forward and back slowly and smoothly and recheck. Did the sides remain even, or did they shift? The movement will get the brain's attention and the self-correction will happen by itself if the rotation is coming from the torso. Try the motion again, sliding along the chair, not lifting the thighs as you slide. This time, include the contralateral movement of the shoulders at the same time. It's how the shoulders would naturally move in opposition to the hips while walking. You may notice that it doesn't feel natural while you're seated, and may feel like a brain teaser for the first few times. The brain usually pairs contralateral motion of the shoulders with the feet instead of with the knees. Try alternating the movement from the feet while sitting and see the difference!

Using that level of focus to slow down and coordinate an unfamiliar action is really beneficial. Enjoy it and see how long it takes your brain to learn it. At the end of the exercise, feel again into a neutral status for the lower body with the spine and notice if any rotation is there in your pelvis. It should be gone now if there was one. If it's coming from the legs or feet it will be easier to correct while standing. This might also help to reset energy levels and effortless posture if you're working at a desk for most of the day. Every collapse of optimal posture is going to send forces down through the matrix that is your skeleton, your tissue, and connective tissues, and fluids in ways that will over time restructure the matrix.

Giving up optimal, upright posture also loads the internal organs, restricts their motion, and in time will impact their function as well. You could be compromising the health of your lungs, heart, stomach, liver, and intestines. These changes can, when tissue and bone become compressed, alter your posture in a ways that some may think is to be expected with age. It isn't necessarily. Once your rib cage drops, you'll find that your pelvis begins to flex, and the senile posture begins to form. Some researchers have found serotonin communication from the spine to the brain influential in scoliosis in some cases, which I find fascinating. Serotonin is present in the periosteum, or outer lining of bone. It has been shown to influence bone metabolism (which affects cognition), the blood, internal organs, immune function, digestion, as well as mood. (Junhua, LV, Feng Liu, *"The Role of Serotonin beyond the Central Nervous System during Embryogenesis,"* Front Cell Neurosci, 2017)

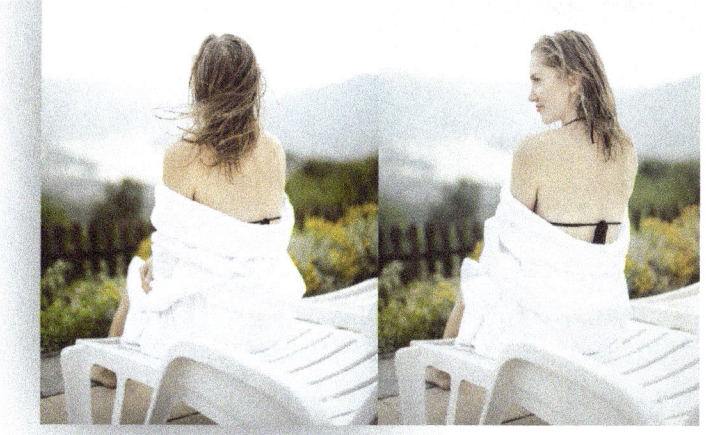

Serotonin could play a role in senile posture as well, which could happen well before old age, but prevention is the key!

## Sitting as a global event

Once your pelvis is resting optimally with the lower legs and bones of the femur, it's the right time to look at the influence of the upper extremities on the spine and the pelvis. The intention will be to integrate the entire body in global perception; sensing it all at the same time. There will be lapses of this global perception during an engaging activity in front of you, unless you make it a point to retain that awareness. It will be a noble venture should you choose to accept this mission, and the rewards will be immeasurable. In any case, if you set up the resting baseline and integrate that experience throughout your body at the outset of sitting, you'll experience an effortless posture and increased energy almost all day long.

While maintaining the awareness and baseline already set up for the lower body, notice your spine as you lift your forearms slowly with palms facing up. Monitor where the change in the extremity is loading the rest of the body. Check in the hips, legs, abdomen, spine, and rib cage. Mind you, there will be extra stabilization support generated in many areas of the body whenever the arms are extended away from the body. So you're initiating an intention to distribute the work of the muscles as evenly as possible. In that vein, scan again and notice where the work may be a little uneven when the palms are facing up, upper arms as relaxed as possible by your sides.

Have your hands empty initially, then experiment with holding a few different items that vary slightly in weight. Compare how it feels up through the fingers and wrists, forearms, biceps, shoulder joint, shoulder girdle, neck, spine, intercostals (between the ribs), and pelvis. Notice if you are gripping slightly in your legs or feet, and if the amount of effort used feels even or unbalanced. Explore holding your hands out by your sides and contrast those sensations with holding them near the midline next to one another. Close your eyes and try both positions again, and re-assess as the sensations become more pronounced. Where are they more pronounced?

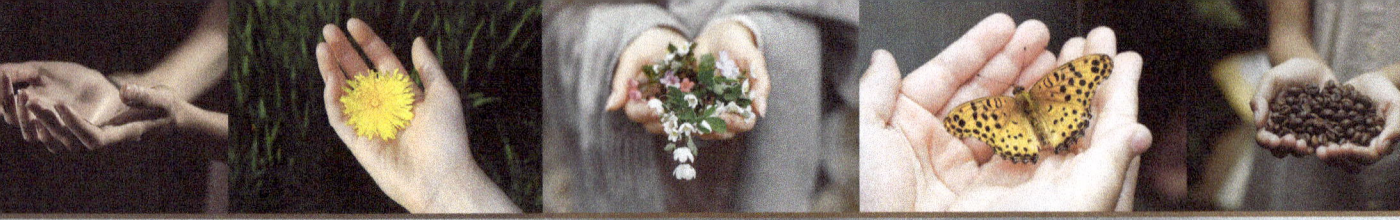

Distinguish whether the work is more in one area or another, or if there are areas that are providing feedback that feels a little dull. Tune into the sensations of the objects you're holding and describe them to yourself in detail. Practice labeling differences. Shift your legs, hips, feet, and torso in whatever ways that help to achieve maximum balance that includes the position and weight of your hands. You may want to bend more or less at the wrist or fingers. Swivel your arms in and out at the elbow to test what difference each position makes. Is there pressure from a jacket or bra on your shoulders? Fan out into global awareness while still monitoring each area. Find out what adjustments can be made in each sector of your body that will optimize your arms feeling weightless as their integration with the rest of your system becomes ideal. Have you discovered neutral everywhere?

Applying this exercise to how you sit at your desk when you're working or to how you drive your car will minimize any strain patterns from cropping up, and will help each activity to happen more smoothly. The attention in your brain is freed up for what you're doing when parts of it don't have to compensate for a tension that is mounting in various places. Just for practice, flip your hands over so that the palms are facing downward like they would be in playing the piano and in so many activities we engage in. The fingers and hands are always engaging the forearm extensors that are connected to them when the palms are facing down.

We're not often working the fingers when our palms are facing up except to hold or carry something. Notice the different effect that this position produces in your forearms and up the chain into the shoulders and into your chest. Therefore, you'll likely feel more dullness and tightness in this position. Move up and find ways to reposition your neck to that your head feels neutral and weightless on top of it. Does balancing your head and neck reduce tension in your hands and arms? Try slowly stretching out your fingers as wide apart as they can go, then gradually bring them back together. Notice which areas between the fingers or between the bones in the hands feel a little tighter than the others.

Hold those places a few seconds longer the next time you expand outward, lifting your shoulders up and down a couple of times. Did you feel the change in your fingers after moving your shoulders? Now, make simultaneous tiny circles with any finger that is tighter than the others and the thumb on that same hand. Practice isolating the finger if it's initially difficult. Then expand the fingers away from one another again and compare from the first attempt. If you don't feel much of a change, curl your fingers, then stretch them upwards a few times and check again.

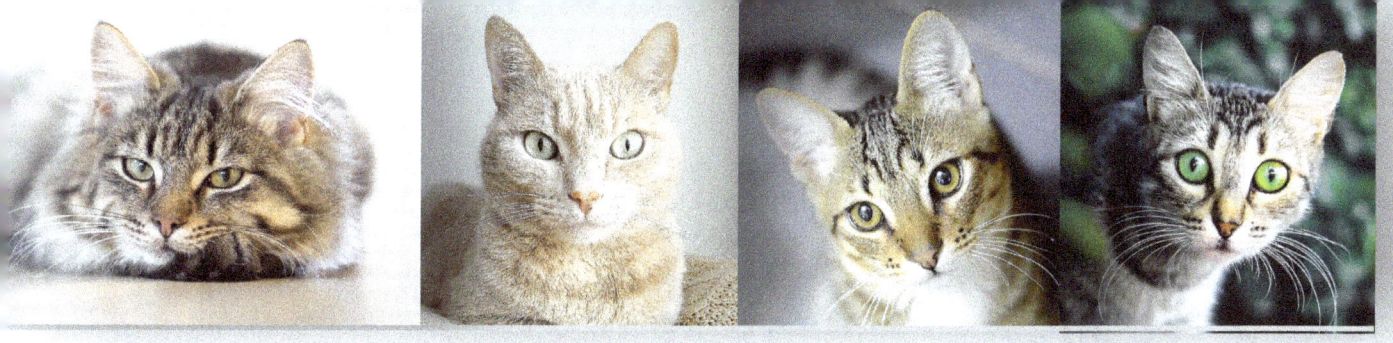

## The eyes have it

The next feature that makes an enormous difference in how relaxed the body will be in any situation is the eyes. They are connected to nearly every experience we will ever have, even while sleeping, and will be paired with countless pathways throughout the brain. In whatever the activity is, particularly if you will be in it for a while, it's a good idea to take a moment to see if you're projecting out with or receiving in with your eyes. The recruitment of muscles will be completely different, as the brain will interpret how you're using your eyes as a cue whether to prepare for action or not.

Take a moment now to see what's happening with your gaze, even while reading. Are you receiving the material or going out to get it with your eyes? Whichever it is, do a scan of your system that has now learned to be globally aware and at rest, then move a piece of your attention to your eyes. Stare out with them and feel which muscles respond immediately to that action. It's a small act, but with a major response from your system. Check the membranes around your skull, jaw, neck, spine, along with the back of your legs as you stare out with your eyes. It's as if your system becomes ready to move forward with all that engagement. Now let your eyes relax and sink back a bit into their sockets and rest. Try to feel the inside of your eyelids.

Notice any changes in tension patterns and once again integrate the local focus into the global whole as you rediscover integration of the eyes with your baseline. By now you should feel like you're floating. You also now have a barometer by which to compare the extent of integration or localized tension in your system. There is such an effortless balance when your system is integrated, that when something is a little bit off, it will stand out like a bullhorn. When the system is balanced, there will be the felt-sense of neutral everywhere. No one area is working harder than it should against gravity, or in place of another area that's working less than normal.

In contrast, when not integrated, your limbs will feel heavier, your eyes will feel more tired, and your posture will begin to sag. There will be many widespread sensations eventually when the forces begin to build up. That will be the language

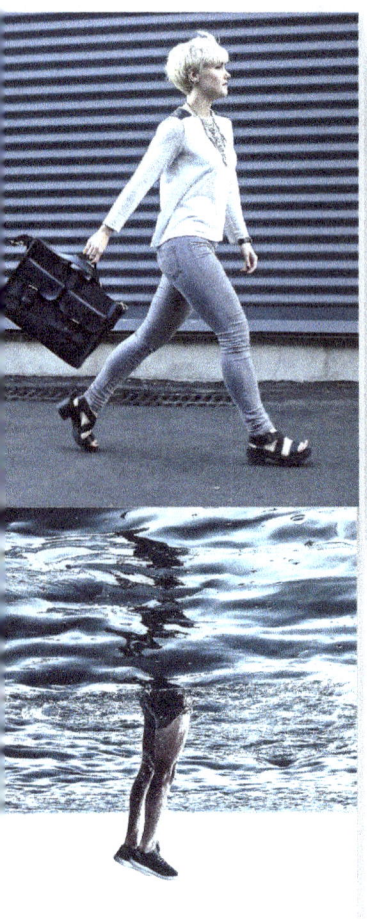

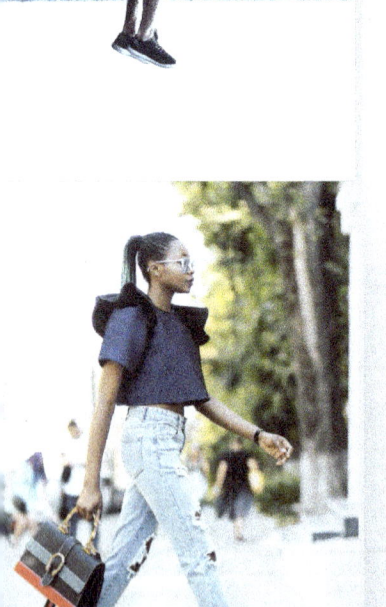

of the body letting you know that it's losing energy and efficiency in the current, imbalanced state of affairs. That's your cue to feel into which area is the most influential in the collapse. It very often will be the feet, center of gravity, or the eyes.

If your neck begins to fatigue you can guess that it has leaned in too far out of alignment with the spine, or your arms are extended out too far away from your body. Although when standing, the neck receives many cues from the feet as to where to position your head; while sitting, that input isn't available so it may drift more easily. In this case, try tapping your feet on the floor slightly to remind your neck where to put your head. When you achieve integration while walking, your stride will feel easy, graceful, and light, as if you were gliding on air with minimal felt sense of your muscles needing to work to carry you along.

If you've maintained the passive, neutral status with your eyes, you might even begin to notice more detail in your surroundings along with brighter, more vibrant colors. In every case, you'll be increasing in awareness, minimizing wear and tear on your system, and maintaining the efficient use of energy throughout the day. You'll also be building a deeper relationship with your body, which will serve you both all of your life. You can apply the same principles of self-sensing when you're standing.

Long hours at a cash register or podium can be taxing on the entire system. The loads will be distributed a little differently when mostly standing still, and the architecture of your feet may shift the forces up the legs and into the hips according to where they are in your feet. Shoes will also have an impact so you will want to compare how it feels with each pair you use, paying special attention to those you will be standing still versus exercising in.

Take notice of how the shoestrings fit across the instep, as those bones and soft tissue fields will be reacting to pressure during a time when you'll be wanting optimal flexibility there. Test the ability of your ankle joint to move freely and whether or not the soles of the shoes you're wearing allow the free motion of the foot with each step you take. If you feel that your foot is a solid block in the shoe, some adjustments may need to be made to keep your feet healthy going forward.

The movement or lack thereof of the feet and ankles will have a tremendous influence on the joints above. Reduced motion could potentially stiffen fascial chains that reverberate all the way up the body into the head. There are minimalist shoes being made these days that have comfort, flexibility, and support, as well as more flexible orthotics if you're in that population that requires them. Unnecessary tension in the arch can lead to plantar fasciitis which is pretty painful and could be preventable when forces are removed from the calf, the arch, and the related connective tissue. We all have internal sensors within our fascia—which surrounds and permeates muscles—that self-regulate according to the external pressures received moment-to-moment.

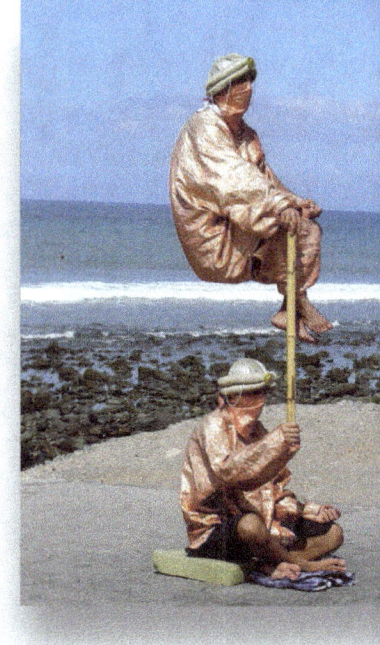

They also remain alert to keep the tissue matrix balanced by its own internal forces while you're changing or maintaining position. (Donald E. Ingber, *"Tensegrity I. Cell structure and hierarchical systems biology,"* Journal of Cell Science, 2003) However, the loads that we apply in daily life occur at a pace that the internal systems cannot reset as quickly as we apply those pressures. Therefore, tuning in to the internal signals that alert you to tensions as they form is key to retaining balance. The overall aim is to achieve a sense of weightlessness as you sit and move through the day, with a balanced distribution of the workload the muscle groups are performing. Ideally, that integration will also be felt in relationship to the objects you come into contact with at work, in vehicles, and at home.

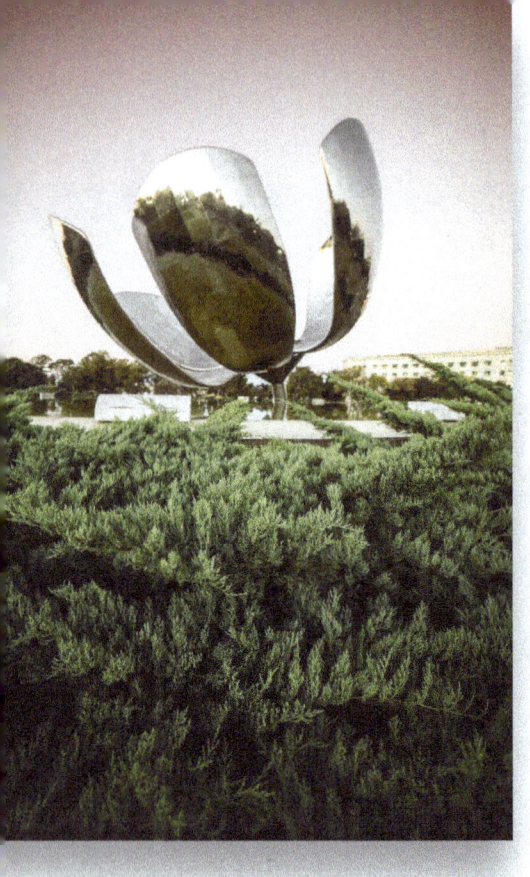

## Chapter 5

## Somatic In-sights (seeing within)

Once you've become accustomed to responding to your body's vocabulary that helps retain physical well-being, you can learn how to go even deeper. You can begin to listen for its cues that also serve on mental, emotional and spiritual levels. The soma is a portal to a host of new, subtle perceptions that cross the bridge from feeling better into healing and wholeness. All it takes is a keen interest in where the intelligence of your body is taking you. Each person's system will have a set of sensory vocabularies that may be specific to your condition, and even that may vary from season to season, and moment to moment, in constant flux.

In this case, healing into wholeness will be gaining awareness of the whole of you; of how the heart, nervous system, biophotons, and energetic systems of your physical form interconnect with the subtle fields around you through your consciousness. Becoming aware of these dynamic relationships can and will reveal their influence upon imbalances and discomforts in your physical body. You may also begin to notice how being out of sync with those subtle fields while being out of touch with consciousness contributes to the lack of well-being. I'll share some of the circumstances that kept enticing me into these more subtle areas that are in full-on communication and interdependence with everything else.

I'm not the only one who's had a fascination with this topic. Several in the fields of quantum physics have been trying to figure out how the Universe expresses its Intelligence. They've known for a while about the ability of one piece of information to be expressed and recognized simultaneously in more than one place at a time. They just aren't sure how. There seems to be some areas of agreement that the 'field' is Conscious, that Consciousness is different from the mind, and that the mind exists outside of the brain. Dr. Karl Pibram, professor of Neuropsychology at

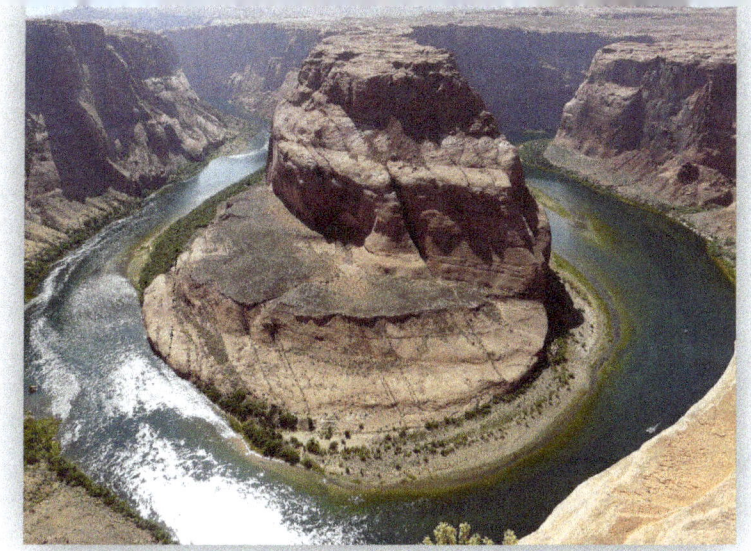

Stanford University finds that, "While during ordinary levels of excitation of the frontolimbic system the signal processing creates the usual narrative consciousness, when the excitation of this system exceeds a certain threshold, conscious experience is dominated by unconstrained holographic processes. The result is timeless, spaceless, causeless, 'oceanic' sensation."

Using an electroencephalograph to measure brain changes, his team noticed that the synchrony created by meditation, prayer, and other relaxation techniques is able to facilitate the 'quantum brain' effect, whereby the individual consciousness becomes linked with the Universal consciousness. According to Pibram, a type of resonance is achieved, similar to strings in a chord being played together, that enables the exchange of information. He demonstrated that, 'receptor fields of cortical neurons" respond, enabling the transduction of information into a form that the individual mind can decode.

Francisco De Biase proposes that, "Our mind is a subsystem of a universal hologram, accessing and interpreting this holographic universe. We are interactive, resonant, and harmonic systems with this unbroken self-organizing wholeness. We are this holoinformational field of consciousness, and not observers to it. The external observer's perspective made us lose the sense and the feeling of unity…" (Biase, "*Quantum Information Self-Organization and Consiousness: A Holoinformational Model of Consciousness*" with Homage to Sir Francis Eccles, Nobel Prize in Medicine) Paradoxically, we are able to use the mirror of the mind to both organize and be organized by this one continuum of Intelligence. Diving into the deeper, more subtle realms of sensing into coherent balance in our systems opens awareness to the larger whole we are receiving information from and expressing information into.

My hope was to be able to understand and be able to perceive the mechanisms that bridged these subtler, energetic, and field-related communication with the physical ones in ways that served health. A few researchers are finding that

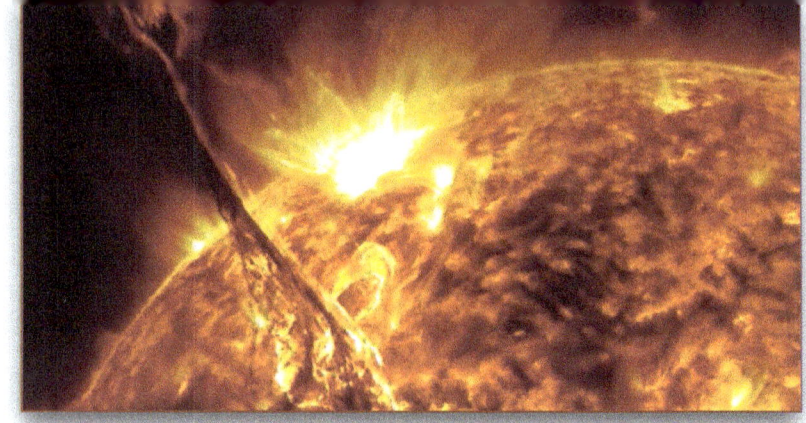

microtubules within the neurons are responsible for receiving and storing information. James Beichler, PhD states, "Within individual neurons, microtubules act as bio-magnetic induction coils that become electromagnetic transceivers in conjunction with axon wall capacitors. They are the primary structural bio-unit used for building, storing, and retrieving memories in the mind." He goes on to say that, *"All cells have similar cell walls (that act as capacitors - something that stores energy in an electrical field) and microtubules can be found in all cells, so very simple and non-complex memory patterns can exist throughout the whole body. So mind and consciousness cannot be limited to the brain alone....The higher complexity level domain structures that constitute higher levels of consciousness can actually guide evolution since each domain level is an organizing agent for lower levels, as is consciousness for mind, and mind for the matter/energy pattern."* (Beichler, "*The Neuro-Cosmological Basis of Consciousness and Spirituality,*" 2013)

From the somatic point of view, gaining self-awareness using conscious movement is the doorway to the more complex, subtle layers. It also facilitates changes that can improve how we function, feel amazing, and increases sensitivity. It enhances the flow of information from the larger fields of Intelligence that guide us and help us to live in sync with the whole of who we are. Current theories about how this continuum between the larger field of influence and our body focuses on the nervous system as the bridge. Subtle structures act as the antennae that pick up the electromagnetic signals and decode them into forms we can understand.

To give you an idea of the scale we're talking about that is processing information into thought forms, the microfilaments that allow glide inside of muscle and nerve cells are 1/1000th the size of a micrometer, which is 1/1000th the size of a millimeter. That's how small nanometers are, which measure the filaments and microtubules we're talking about. Energies can be stored, according to Beichler, in microtubules which are between 8-25nm long. The fact that they form a spiral increases their storage capacity. Garaiev, a Russian researcher, noticed that biophotons act preferably upon the cell nucleus where DNA resides. The implication is then that light particles are transmitting information that is affecting how your entire body functions, and our thoughts merge with light particles.

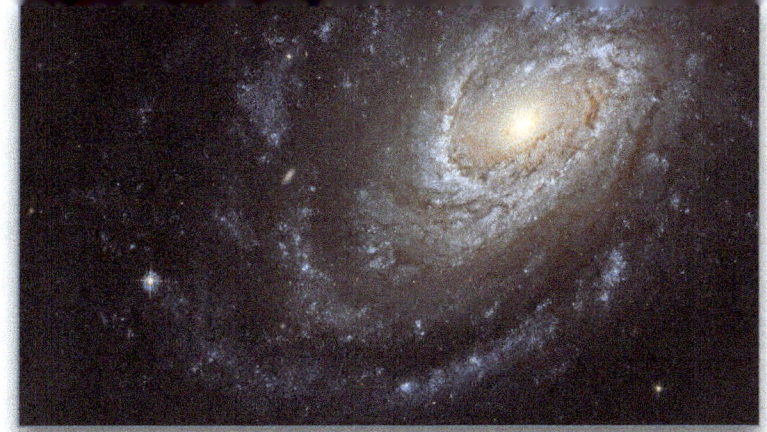

I've wondered whether the energetic systems are participating as a bridge between the larger field and the nervous system, both of which connect into all other systems. There are several different types of energy systems and I've only studied four of them: Polarity, Chi, Primo Vascular, and Nadis, which connect with Marmas. The primo vascular system interconnects with literally every other system in the body and delivers energy forms that are biochemical, like adrenaline, ATP, ADP, glucose, and water. It also carries neurotransmitters, hormones, amino acids, hyaluronic acid, and nucleotides. The chi that flows through meridians and points according to Chinese acupuncture is believed to be connected with certain nerve cells and internal organs, along with other systems and their functions. Various chi kung practices involve sending, receiving, circulating and storing chi which have proven beneficial effects for the body.

## Entering the deep body

As sensing abilities increase, it is possible to assess the flow along meridians and its connection to symptoms. If you're wondering whether or not it's possible to sense something so tiny, just think that most acupuncturists can sense meridians, which are about 15um (micrometers) wide. A human hair is about 75 microns wide. At some point along the way in my sequence of concussions and differentiating the type, location, and cause of the set of painful symptoms that arose, I felt restrictions in certain meridians that were beginning to hurt. In some cases, the sensation followed the path of a nerve, but the diversions revealed that it had its own trajectory. For example, the "Are You Kidding Me?" head bang on the wall after the exercise ball rolled out of control, followed the paths of the Governing Vessel, the Bladder meridian all the way into the foot, and certain parts of the Triple Heater meridian in the head. It also captured parts of the sciatic nerve and the descending nerve pathways from the motor cortex.

During the spatial orientation and vestibular phases, it's easy to be off balance and have another mishap. This was true a few months after the ball incident, when I miscalculated where the freezer door was while it was open, and bumped the side

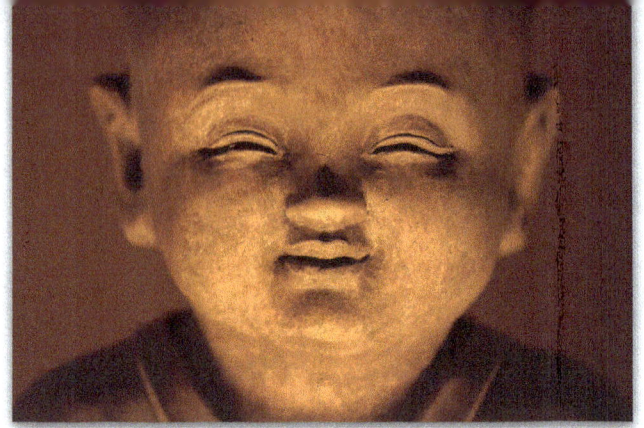

of my head ever so slightly. When you've had dozens of head injuries however, a slight tap can send the brain reeling. Hence the motivation to erase the cumulative effects of prior injuries as much as possible was keen. Do keep this in mind if you think to tell yourself, "It was barely a tap! It couldn't be from that."

The happy surprise is that much of the investigation and reorganization that happened between the ball incident and the freezer mishap 6 months later showed that indeed the latter one was nearly a stand-alone episode, but triggered an old broad-side car accident where my head bounced off the window. Most of the symptoms were contained on the left side of the body, beginning with locking up the temporal bone, area, restricting blood flow under the collar bone, and over-stimulating the area of the sensory-motor cortex related to the eyes and the hands. It affected everything on the left side from head to toe.

This sensation was odd—not like nerve pain or numbness—but more like the Velcro stickiness that burns a little when fascia becomes glued. Glued to what? It twisted my cervical spine again as it yielded to the deformations of the membranes inside the skull. I learned from prior injuries that this type of 'shock' impact tension doesn't respond well to fluid intervention when the membranes are that stuck. It's best to head for fascial and vascular restrictions and unstick them first to increase mobility, and make space for fluid flow. The temporal bone moved easily again by freeing energy in the gall bladder and triple heater meridians in the head.

The Gall Bladder and Small Intestine meridians were irritated, each of which benefited from opening the entire length of the pathway. The cervical spine responded well after a few somatic reminders. Muscles alongside the spine were compromised mostly due to the altered curvature in the neck, and they, along with the rotator cuff were happy to release when the neck resumed its normal position. Gently opening the sticky sheath around the vagus nerve eased abdominal sensitivities, which drew me once again to the umbilical hernia scar. A tiny bit more adjustment inside the navel freed a slight, internal restriction that pretty much eliminated the lower abdominal gastric reactions. This seemed like the perfect opportunity to investigate further into the more subtle areas to see if they were carrying some of the shock. In the Hindu traditions some of the major chakras, or

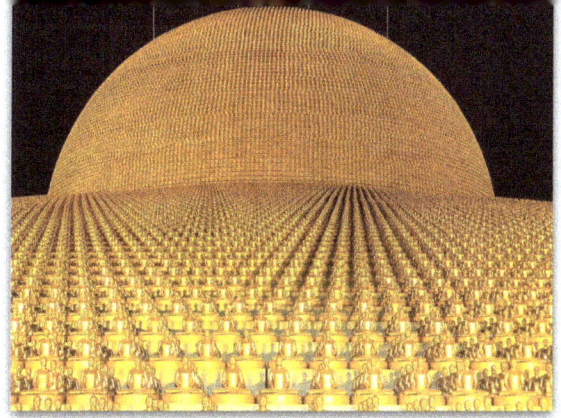

energy centers in the body, correspond to major nerve plexus. One of my teachers mentioned that nerve plexus often capture shock to prevent it from landing in the brain or in nearby organs. Energetic systems are also related to the fields surrounding the body, so I decided to investigate there.

## Biophotons

Biophotons, which circulate both in and around the body, have been shown to reflect the status of coherence in the system. They also interact with the nervous system. A 2011 study reports that, "Neural cells also continuously emit biophotons. The intensity of biophotons is in direct correlation with neural activity, cerebral energy metabolism, EEG activity, cerebral blood flow and oxidative processes. (Rahnama, et. al., *"Emission of Mitochondrial Biophtons and Their Effect on Electrical Activity of Membranes via Microtubles"*, Journal of Integrative Neuroscience, Vol. 10, No.1, 2001) I wondered which of these systems was creating these new sights and sounds in and around my brain, and was excited to find out. They also mentioned the possible correlation between biophotons and Alpha brainwave activity—which I'd tested to have high amounts of—and can also affect sleep patterns.

In answer to the question of whether or not biophotons can be a source of cellular communication, researcher Sergey Mayburov says, "The answer is that it does," he says. "Biophoton streams consist of short quasi-periodic bursts, which he says are remarkably similar to those used to send binary data over a noisy channel." Mayburov noticed the ability of cells to use non-local communication to sync up growth patterns in eggs. The author goes on to say, "That might help explain how cells can detect such low levels of radiation in a noisy environment. Mayburov likens this form of communication to the way error-correcting software sends binary data over a noisy incoherent channel." (MIT Technology Review, May 2012)

As early as the 1970s Fritz Popp and his researchers were able to determine that, "The biophotons emitted from our cells are highly coherent energy that may be responsible for the operation of our living systems." Coherence implies a highly

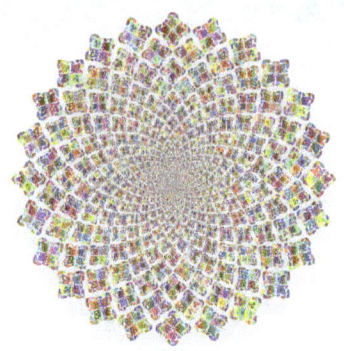

structured, organized frequency. Russian scientist Peter Garaiev found that after infusing DNA in a tube with a laser, a form of highly coherent light, the DNA absorbed the light, which then replicated the exact spiral of the DNA's helix. The light retained the imprint of the spiral even after the DNA was removed, leaving the researchers in a quandary as to what was holding the shape in place. The team speculated that the light was probably connected to an external source that was able to record and retain the impression. I have indeed seen, that a space, and even objects, retain the information of prior experiences. There is apparently an underlying implicate order that retains the formation in the space, like a memory, the way that our subtle bodies do.

It appears that there are external forces dynamically related to this form of light, and that cellular function and communication is not just a by-product of molecular processes. Other experiments have shown that these fields of light can be influenced and enhanced by us, and are related to the health of the organism emitting the biophotons. After the Human Genome Project found in 2012 that only 1% of our DNA (over 20,000 genes) translates into a traceable protein, the rest was classified as 'junk' DNA. However, it had already been discovered by Harvard biologists and linguists in 1994 that the nucleotide bases of this so-called 'junk' DNA express all of the features of language. They include syntax, semantics, and grammar, calling it 'wave genetics'. (Flam, 1994) There is every likelihood that we can and do participate in this language unconsciously. As thoughts connect to biophotons, we surely do participate, so making it conscious is transformative.

Going back even further, cellular interactions were noticed by Gurswitsch in 1926 and 1934 in onions, later reproduced by plants which have also been shown to signal one another non-physically. Later studies on the subject revealed that "photosensitive biomolecules of cells and neurons can absorb and transmit photons, and transfer the absorbed biophoton energy to nearby biomolecules by resonance energy transfer, which can induce conformation changes and trigger complex signal processes in cells and between cells" (Sun Y., 2010). More research is on the way to further understand the role of light in the transmission of information throughout the body, which mainly seems to happen via our DNA, but it remains clear that it is a language that the body uses to communicate.

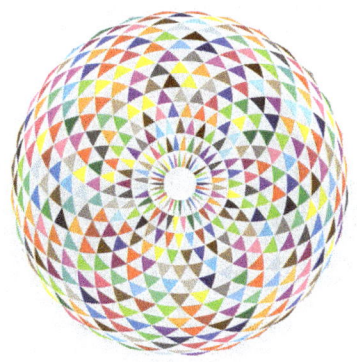

In his article on the subject, (*6th Sense: Are We Communicating Using Invisible Light? Biophotons and DNA.*") Dr. Michael Kana goes on to say, "Biophotons could offer that supplementary signaling pathway next to electrical and chemical pathways for intra- and intercellular communication" (Popp & Zhang, Mechanism of interaction between electromagnetic fields and living organisms, 2000; Shen, Mei, & Xu, 1994). I believe that the implications are vast by allowing in the influence of these subtler levels of communication as significant factors in the diagnosis and treatment of disease as well as for the maintenance of health.

Curiosity in the middle of the night when certain energetic changes in the field woke me up again and again even when not in pain, led me to question the changes in the patterns of the light particles I was seeing in the room. Mind you, they are also present everywhere outside, but those particles in the room have proven to be more reflective of what's happening in my own system rather than in nature. That said, there is a tremendous burst of them in the field every sunrise as every life form receives that energy/frequency. Biodynamic training naturally led me to be oriented towards coherence in the fluid field, and other teachers had mentioned that trauma can be stored as memory in the field surrounding the body. I was stoked to explore the possible reflections in the field of my system, and my ability to influence these light particles.

## Increasing coherence

This curiosity led me to compare what was happening in the field from day to day, using coherence as a value to compare changes with. Then I'd consider the status of my body before bed: i.e. what I'd eaten, what my brain felt like, if I'd had a cardiovascular workout that day, where I'd been, how long using electronics, etc. I logged how the field looked and felt depending upon the day's activities, then began to explore the possibility of changing the field using various approaches. There were so many notable relationships that I won't list them all here, but suffice to say that using methods to increase coherence had a great, immediate influence on my system. My body was indeed listening to this form of communication. There were many, many factors affecting the activity in the field that were generating a more chaotic pattern, but it didn't take many methods to return the field to balance.

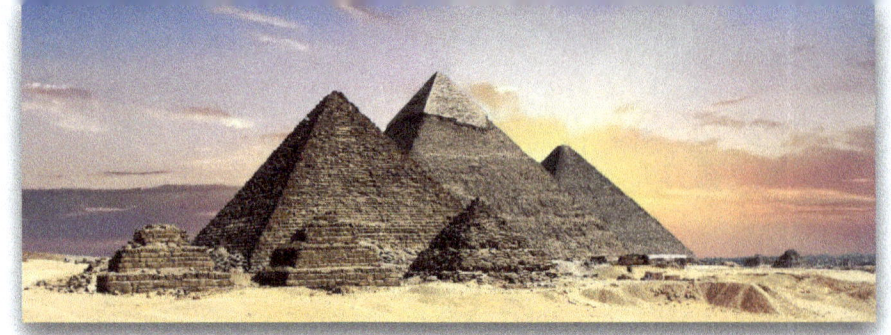

Looking more closely did reveal five main factors: daily experiences affected the coherence of the field through the way my muscles, fluids and joints felt, the status of internal organs and physiology, mental and emotional state, and energetic status. Having had so many head injuries, I would naturally lean towards checking cranial/brain issues first, but it more often was those unresolved issues that created unrest in the field. Issues not fully resolved also generated aches and pains in my system. Those subconscious residues couldn't be held back during sleep; the stuff that dreams are made of. I wondered if maintaining a calm, neutral state all day would retain the coherence at night. That was true for many years when life was simpler and the mind was more quiet!

As some researchers have alluded to, biophotons are a form of communication that interact with neurons. Waiting quietly while tuning in to them will usually reveal the thoughts that are lingering and still manifesting in the field. 'Listening' to the light particles usually brought solutions in almost immediately. Light is a form of electromagnetic communication, so other electromagnetic interactions could also impact the field. One consistent aggravator to the field would be too much time on a cell phone or in front of the computer, especially in the evening. It would either strain the mucous membranes of the sinuses or the eyes or both. Overstimulating the nervous system through sound also fatigued it and created irritation that was reflected in the field.

Sacred geometry is a language that light particles recognize, so it seemed logical to try using those shapes to influence the field. They helped normalize frequencies coming off of the electronics, and helped protect my body from them as well. A pyramid helped every time. Other balanced patterns like the Flower of Life, Merkabah (tetrahedron), platonic solids, the cross, a three-dimensional cross that I was shown in a dream, and other mandalas can and do help to reorganize the field back into a coherent form. Many reports of healing and even calmed weather patterns happen within and around a pyramid constructed according to the Golden Ratio (proportional relationships of sides =1: 1.618 approximately).

The architectural concept of tensegrity—balancing tension created by various forces—applied to our bodies, has been found to show that everything, including our bones, responds to tension and compression according to geometric shapes. *"At the other end of the scale on a micro level, proteins and other key molecules*

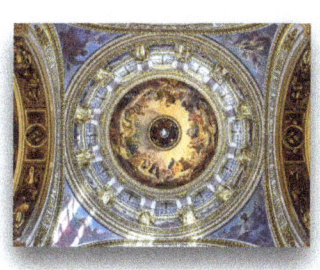 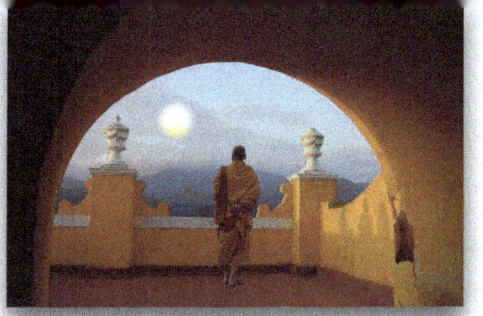 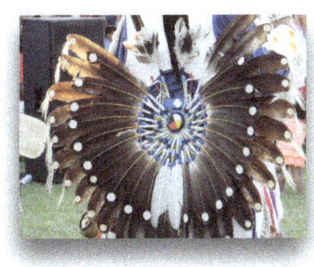

*stabilize through tensegrity. At any scale we wish to view, the body exhibits the same structural building blocks: spirals, pentagons, and triangles."* (Dr R. Paul Lee, *"Interface, Mechanisms of Spirit in Osteopathy,"* 2005) Very little has been explored using these physical laws as forms of interaction that can help the soma to recalibrate, but hopefully it will become more prominent in the future. Mandalas, and Yantras have been used in the East for millennia with Egypt and Greece not far behind. The phenomena of the influence of mathematical patterns aren't new, but not often passed on from Ancient traditions or used for healing. This is probably some of the stuff folks who stumble upon Mystery Schools while traveling in Tibet learn as an initiate, but isn't meant to become common knowledge.

I didn't know where to start to be able to understand what I was seeing and feeling. I'd felt the most comfortable with mystical phenomena in Native American ceremonies because I knew that this, the African, and the Irish part of my heritage have a long history of multi-dimensional experiences. It did seem to be surfacing again, and the ancestral orientation helped me to remain open to enquire and try to learn more about these phenomena. I also noticed that there is a memory in the immediate field—like an Akashic record (a repository on the non-physical mental plane of every thought, action, emotion, of every person in the past, present, and future)—of everything that happens to us. If the subtle fields around my body were waking up in certain ways, it makes sense that some Ancient impressions would begin to surface. This is possibly what drew me to India in the first place. It seemed that all kinds of impressions in the field can become reinvigorated under certain triggers or circumstances.

In any case, it often felt like ancient traditions and ancestral wisdom were the best places to find answers. Many indigenous traditions - Native American, South and Central American, or Aboriginal - see spiritual healing being needed to resolve emotional or physical conditions. Each layer of the subtle bodies expresses in different ways according to East Indian traditions. Some traditions describe the layers as being the physical body, the etheric or trauma imprint layer, the astral, or second emotional layer with emotional imprints, the mental body with soul imprints, and the causal body with spiritual information from the Higher Self. Some say we interact most with the astral layer during sleep. That makes sense with my experience, because this field becomes very alive in the middle of the night, as if those impressions are trying to sort themselves out.

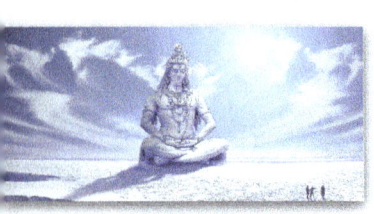 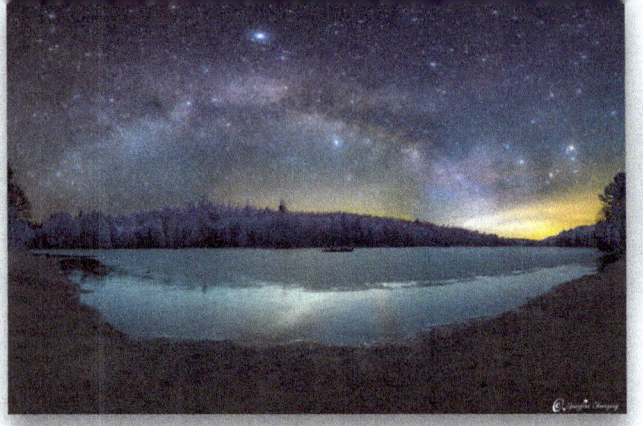 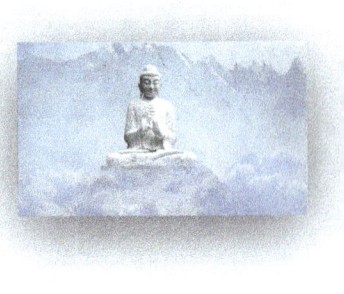

Koshas ('sheaths') is the term from the Upanishads in the Ancient Hindu tradition that yoga is based upon that describes the subtle bodies. The sheaths include: 1) the Annamayakosha/food body; our physical body, 2) Pranamayakosha/energy body, 3) Manomayakosha/mental body, 4) Vijnanamayakosha or wisdom layer, and 5) Anandamayakosha, which is the bliss body where love, peace, and joy reside. Some systems teach that these layers exist separately, and some say that they overlap. One approach will have the outermost layer as the finer layer, another will have the higher, finer layer as residing deep within. Some approaches will have the denser layers sandwiched in between the subtlest layers at the periphery, and the innermost layer. I guess you have to pick a system, experiment with it, and see how the fields within and around you respond.

I experienced the field in both ways. There was a bliss layer deep within as well as a fine (Spirit) outermost layer that both help to clear, settle, transmute, and harmonize perturbations in the middle (mental/emotional) layers. There was no need to understand exactly what was happening to cause the chaos in the middle field for it to settle. However, the nervous system settled more if the related thought processes vibrating in the middle layers were perceived. Releasing and balancing the field enabled light to produce more light, but that wasn't getting at the sticky memories that were keeping the injuries from healing all the way.

Daily experiences created little tension areas all over my body, whether from physical exertion, sensory stimulation, or mental/emotional activation. This also happens through the nervous system and meridians, where the restrictions create discomfort, soreness, and tension. Imbalances and restrictions could prolong healing, but there was something more specific that was the missing link for the head injuries. While waiting to discover those specific connections, I found other ways to cohere the field and feel better besides contemplating the subtle bodies.

Prayer, or invoking a Divine presence, works beautifully. Resting in that presence as it blesses, uplifts, balances, forgives, redeems, and releases the impressions is transformative. If there are deeper, subconscious impressions that are attaching themselves to the injury patterns, the light of awareness will need to reveal why they are there for the healing to be complete. Otherwise, the pattern will be

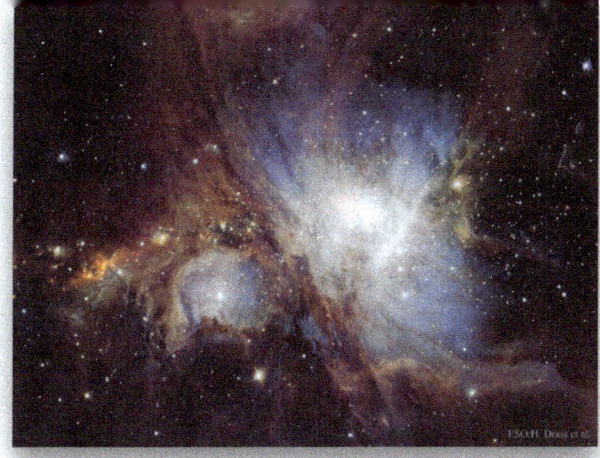

vulnerable to returning and creating the same issues again with the right trigger. Sticky bits can be sitting in the subtle fields just as they can in various layers in the physical form.

I believe that these old traumas situated in the 'aches and pains' we feel, or in the fields around the physical body, are what wind up creating illnesses, anxiety, depression, and you name it. That's the difference between 'feeling better' and healing. You can go to a yoga class and stretch, get some bodywork, meditate, have a drink, take some meds, or what have you to feel better and take care of those day-to-day stressors. However, if the deeper memories and impressions are not released or reorganized, dysfunctions of many varieties will most likely be the prognosis. Realizing that there are very microscopic places that contain these memories will be of enormous value in your ability to access healing.

The desire to heal all the way is a big part of being able to access everything you need to. Once the subconscious 'no' and reasons to avoid those traumas are out of the way, half the battle is already won. Also, when you make contact with the subtle layers of your being, you've gone past the physical, mental, and emotional layers into the wholeness of who you are. When you're more identified with your Spirit than with your experiences, the healing will be faster, easier, and more complete. Even if karmas, or consequences of past actions, may be a factor in things attaching—waiting for their receipts to get cashed in—Grace is always present for forgiveness and redemption to help mitigate those consequences.

When enough resting balance and integration have happened so that the inner core is shining the light of love, joy, and bliss from Anandamayakosha into them, they are already transformed. They wouldn't be able to create misery or negative feelings ever again. It's helpful to contemplate or meditate until you feel that those particles are exiting the heart, enabling its fire to begin to permeate, purify, and liberate. You may not sense 'particles' per se, leaving you. You may just feel lighter, more spacious, and an impulse to take a deep breath; like a weight has been lifted, or a door that had been closed just opened.

 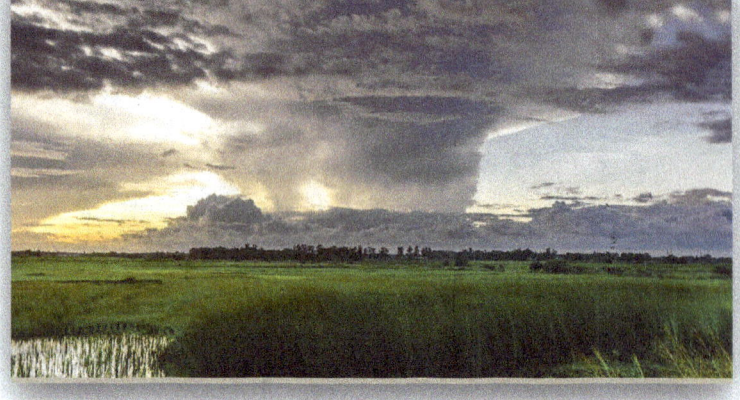 

## The eye of a storm in an injury

Suffice to say, what we are is a very complex system that works intricately together in miraculous ways. When you've made it a practice to become more familiar with the vocabulary your body uses to communicate, you'll be guided into the system that needs the attention. When you get to that system, it's best to find the calm center being the fulcrum, before trying to correct it. In my case, it was often my eyes and ears that were still overly sensitive from old head injuries. If I'd been using the computer for a few hours, or had been on the phone several times, the particles from those devices and the stimulation of energy and nerves was pronounced. Many sensitive people I know experience the same thing.

They pretty much will all stop electronic device use early in the evening, and avoid phone conversations after a certain time. I do the same. In any case, it was clear that other sensory input, along with mental and emotional states at the time had also become tied into the injuries. An entire series of events may have become stitched together somehow in the overlapping subtle bodies and nadis. A Spiritual teacher, H.W.L. Poonja, whom we affectionately called Papaji, spoke about the four horses that drag you away from Truth. Those four horses were the senses. The senses convince us that experiences are more real than our deeper Nature. One experiences are identified with by the personality, our bodies don't really understand how to process them without guidance. So the memories with charge on them wind up in cellular storage, waiting for instructions on how to proceed. In the meantime, those stored, confused experiences kick up a storm on the surface of your body.

We then adopt all sorts of routines (yoga, jogging, chiropractic, alcohol, etc.) to discharge the discomfort resulting from all that we take in, but the loop continues to run. By middle age most folks feel pretty compromised in their health. I sure did. Feeling better may be similar to transcending the 'pain body' that Eckhart Tolle

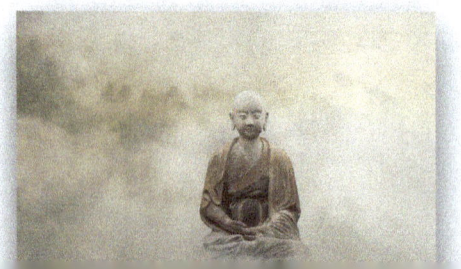

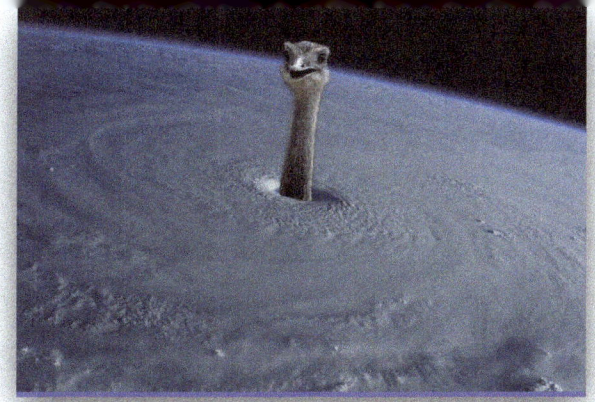

speaks about where certain unseemly parts of us become disembodied and reside in the emotional body surrounding the physical one. This 'pain body' may be equivalent to the etheric/emotional, energy, and astral bodies spoken of in Ancient texts. Tolle discusses how those energetic forces from the unconscious can appear like 'demons' we must face, or ego patterns that are resistant to surrendering to the light within. Those patterns put up a fight in a variety of ways that can be so disturbing and confusing, that you may prefer to keep them repressed.

Even meditation can be a way to get around facing them directly. I experienced years of blissful meditations and satoris that made daily life challenges seem like a breeze that love could always overcome. This was after years of therapeutic practices that seemed to have resolved early traumas. Yet at night, there would be this light show in my room that I assumed was coming from the more recent head injuries. When I realized that remaining in a calm, neutral place brought coherence to those light particles, and that my body responded by releasing tension and pain, I felt I was really on to something significant. And I was, but there was still more.

I only learned after the bump on the freezer door that many, many impressions were still there in those middle subtle layers, even while seeming that my physical, energetic, mental and emotional states were in good shape. The fact that they began vibrating at night trying to find resolution was the body's way of letting me know that something subconscious was still unresolved. The attention I paid to the biophotons began to increase. I began to associate the areas in my body that held a sensation, to the area of the field that was behaving erratically. At some point I realized that the intelligence of the light itself was pointing to the area of restriction, over and over again. I didn't need to search for them.

You'd be surprised how disconcerting light phenomena can be when you do feel it, so committing to being the calm in the eye of the storm was really needed. I knew that the heart emitted light and had a huge electromagnetic reach, so I wondered if it was responsible for the erratic patterns in the field. My heart was doing such a

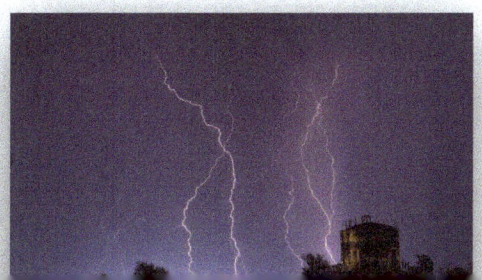

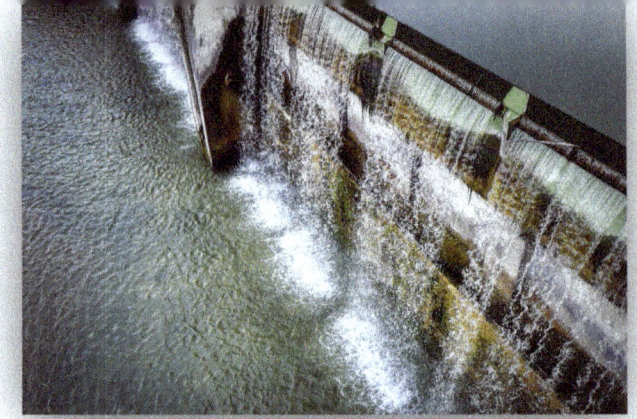

funny dance then—pounding, racing, skipping a beat—that I went to see a cardiologist and had some tests done. He gave my heart a clean bill of health. Even though I wasn't focusing on my heart at the time, while sitting still and tuning in to inner stillness, I saw many old experiences exit my heart in very subtle forms that could only be called energy particles, yet no images or memories came with them. I guess they represented something I was subconsciously holding on to.

## Being your own detective

I wondered if old shocks and injuries prevented daily life experiences from passing through easily, even if you weren't particularly identified with them. There were many questions that needed answering, but it felt best to start from the injuries I knew about, and assume that they weren't all the way healed. Even though they felt better, I needed to dig a little deeper into what was still creating a storm. I followed my hunch that something was off in the vein that poured into my heart. I sensed it right after the injury, and even went for hyperbaric oxygen treatments, but something was still off. There was a major shift in symptoms after I took a vascular class where we manually opened restrictions in the arteries of the upper body.

In fact, the symptoms mostly went away. After that a new type of integration entered my system. There was a smoothing out of the light around my body like I'd not seen in years. It was deeply relaxing and relieving, however I still held a curiosity about the superior vena cava above the right atrium of the heart. Old injuries were expressing barely noticeable signs that would be easy to ignore, and difficult to identify. I just had a hunch there was something going on in the vascular system, and wanted to follow that hunch anyway since a few family members developed conditions in that system that were life-altering.

There were other lingering signs of discomfort from the freezer bump all down the left side that needed attention. There was a nagging sense that woke me up each night of an incessant electrical activity that was out of balance in my brain. Lying down on my face, neck and head while a head injury is trying to heal is always a little tenuous. Each night produced a bit of strenuous pressure that aggravated and

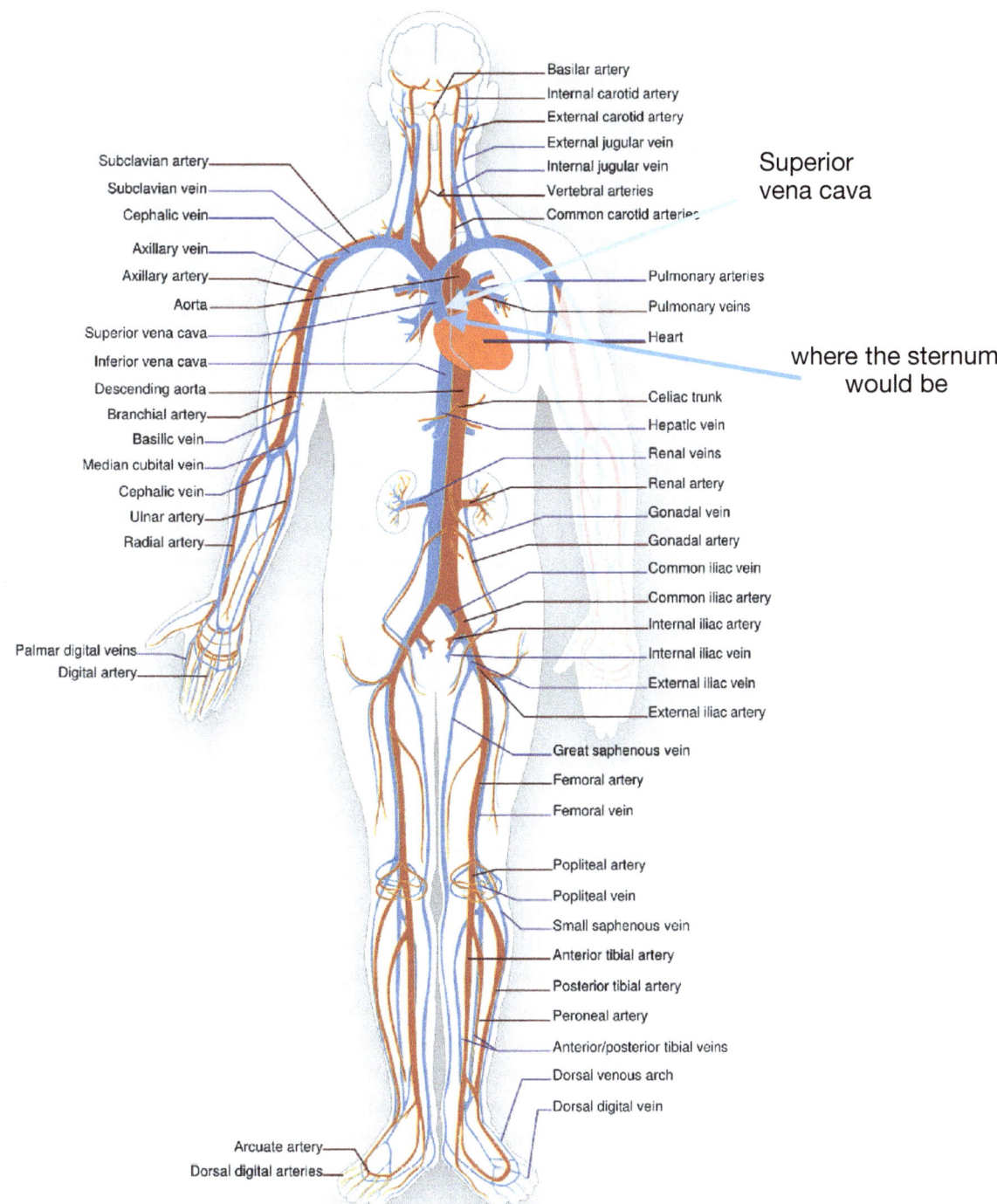

slowed down its ability to heal. Certain tensions were still in the cervical muscles, but history has shown that membranes and other structures inside the skull were likely to be involved. (Remembering earlier communication from your body will be helpful in solving current issues.) Since the base of my skull still felt tight, I checked the upper cervical area, my eyes and their sockets, inside my mouth, my sacrum, and anywhere else I could think of that might be related to the tension there. The sound had some features of tinnitus, but it was located slightly behind the ears, so

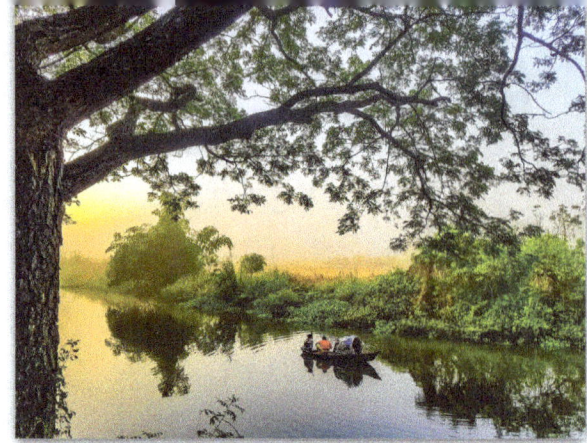

I had to keep looking. It could be from compression in the sutures; in particular, the occipitomastoid suture (page 110) right behind the ears.

There were some catch places around the sternum and upper ribs and collar bone, where some of the anterior neck muscles attached, which also attach near that same area. The tenderness there brought other vascular issues into consideration. Nearly every female client I've worked on had tenderness in the same area, which is right in front of the thymus. I wasn't sure how to interpret that fact, but wanted to return to restrictions in fluid flow that accompany menopause as a possibility. This was also an area where the lymphatic vessels drained into the heart for release through the bloodstream. Congestion in that fluid system could also create soreness. Soreness in middle-aged women who attempt to gain more upper body strength is very common. Even yoga tightens this same area in women.

The familiar sensation of Velcro stickiness with a slight burn to it was in those areas and I decided to check for myofascial restrictions around the walls of the arteries or veins A teacher once described the sensation that veins produce as being electrical, so I wondered if this electrical 'storm' was being created by congestion in the veins at night limiting the glymphatic system from doing its job to drain waste from the brain. There was an immediate 'yes' from the system as the restrictions in the walls of the brachiocephalic artery, superior vena cava, and aortic arch began to unwind and support the motion through the jugular vein as well as blood flow to the lungs, abdomen, and pelvic bowl. Follow the 'yes'!

At some point I could feel the vascular releases around the collar bone begin to have an impact all the way down through the legs as my calves began to release. I was drawn back to the sternum to check if there was another similar velcro sensation and there was, near the entry to the heart's atrium. These were leftovers from earlier impacts (martial arts, car accidents) but were exacerbated by the recent ones. After checking further, it turns out a few ribs were out of place and my diaphragm was tight as a result. Also, no doubt the phrenic nerve in my neck that innervates the diaphragm had been irritated by both recent cranium impacts, so there were several sources of long-held tension in my chest cavity.

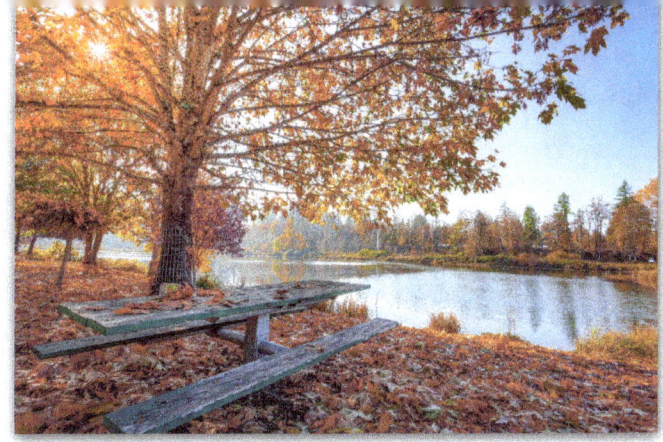

After I'd cleared many of these vascular restrictions, the fineness of the coherence in the field was unmatched. The electrical buzz that sounded similar to tinnitus abated. Maybe the nerves needed inflow from the arteries to calm down. For a brief period, the particles in the field turned into a large, harmonious, peaceful waveform. Theoretical physicist, Dr. David Bohm, views the particle aspect of consciousness as carriers of information. He states, "Electromagnetic energy (such as light or heat) does not always behave in a continuous wave - rather it is grainy because energy can be transferred only in quantum packages. Therefore, light has a dual character. Under certain circumstances, it may display wavelike aspects; and in other circumstances, it may have the characteristic of particles."

When I read that, it seemed like the particles might be a manifestation of an increase in mental activity rather than, or created by the brain injury. However, it makes sense that increased mental activity also increases neural activity. The dots were beginning to connect. Trauma, mental activity, and new information from life transitions could all play a part. The many changes happening out in life and within, could all be reflected in the subtle phenomena; especially if they literally were anatomically connected. The fields around the body were thankfully revealing their language. Developing sensitivity to these areas was well worth the effort.

Let's try some practices that may help you to notice some of the dynamism in the subtle fields of activity, then see if you can notice an influence anywhere in your body. We see so many images internally when we dream or day dream. What's happening within when you're not dreaming? When you close your eyes, your consciousness is seeing something, as well as the sensory apparatus inside your brain. Practice focusing on the little differences you notice inside with your eyes closed. Try picturing a rose, or a strawberry, and notice the field that the strawberry is floating in. Describe any details you see, no matter how small. Is the field solid, or does it have some breaks in it? Is it one color, several shades of one color, or several colors? Which color or pattern do you see? Is there anything that makes the color change that is related to how you hold your head, which image you use, or thoughts you have? See if you can begin to make associations with all of this.

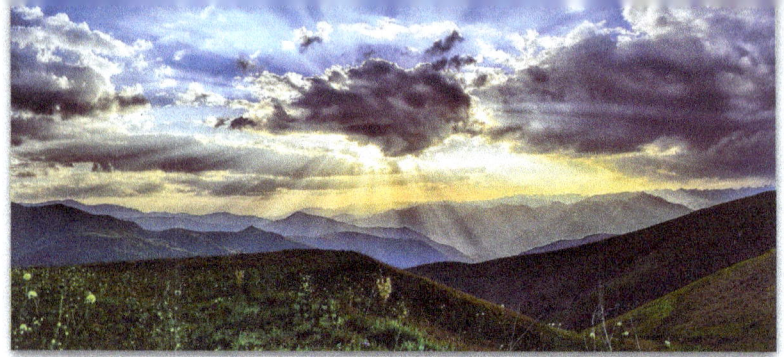

## Connecting the dots along the continuum

I used to see peaceful, translucent or clear light that moved in a slow, entrancing pattern. At that time I viewed it as the 'Sat' or Truth part of Satchitananda, Chit, or the Consciousness aspect was reduced, while the bliss of Ananda was merged into the being aspect. Now it seems the Chit aspect is predominant, and the calm, Sat aspect is not. It's challenging to find the most accurate perspective to interpret the change with. I wanted the light to return to its status as a wave because it had expressed like that for most of my spiritual life. During the explorations in volume 6, after clearing deep tensions and nerve irritations in my neck, the clarity of the light in a waveform returned, bringing in a global calm along with it. Could it be that injuries created restrictions in my neck that interfered with the subtler light being expressed throughout consciousness? I needed to investigate this more.

There was a lot to learn about consciousness, the brain, the heart, the mind, the subtle bodies, biophotons, and their source. Healing my brain would surely prove or disprove one of the theories. I'm leaning towards the light particles reflecting increased activation in my nervous system. That said, the brain, vascular system, energy system, and biochemistry all interact with the nervous system. The next morning the buzz had returned along with the tight, stingy sensation along the left side of my body. Tuning into the origin of the sensation revealed an energetic pulsation at the temple that went deep into that region in the side of my brain. It lifted out several inches from my head, then snapped back as if there was an energetic rubber band pulling it back in place.

I interpreted that as the force vector of the fridge impact still being in the subtle fields. It reverberated back into my nervous system, brain nuclei, and soft tissue. The adjacent blood vessels also reacted along with an additional restriction in the nerve plexus in the face anterior to the jaw. There were a few methods I learned to remove shock from the energy fields in and around the body, so I tried a few of them. It may not seem like much, but banging your head against a hard object is like striking a gong with your brain against your skull. It echoes through the tissue and vibrates through many cells and fluids. I paired the line of shock in the field with the sound and sensations inside

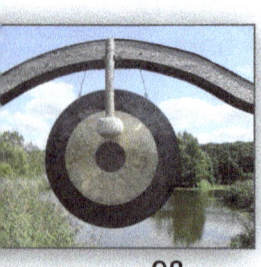

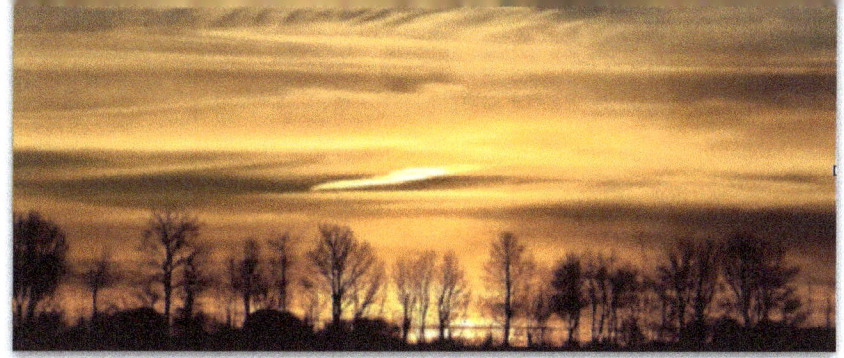

my head until they balanced each other out and silenced.

Dr. Mae Won Ho, a biologist and researcher, finds that the water in our fascia and nerves can also act as superconductors, like crystals. In that sense, and also on a physiological level, it's helpful to tune into the fluid systems within other systems from time to time and make sure they're clear of restriction. In the case of impact injury, the cells' ability to communicate would be greatly altered across pathways that are still shimmering with shock. By increase the somatic vocabulary you use, either by enhanced sensing abilities, or by the expanding upon the structures you're intending to contact, the system will respond in a new way. It will open new areas of balance and integration; each with its own rewards, each taking you a few steps closer to full healing.

Losing awareness is going to happen when you're a busy person with a full plate most of the time. I was learning that what got past my awareness during the day was sitting in the field waiting to be processed in the middle of the night. I decided to use that clear wave of light with the blue pulsation as a goal or signal that my brain had healed, or that my nervous system was settled. The input coming in through the eyes and ears in particular, but also through the mouth could produce an enormous amount of stimulation and activation of the mind. I had noticed that conversations with eye contact were the most stimulating for my brain, and most difficult for sleep unless it was settled out before bed. When you realize that those structures take up half of the sensorimotor cortex, it makes sense.

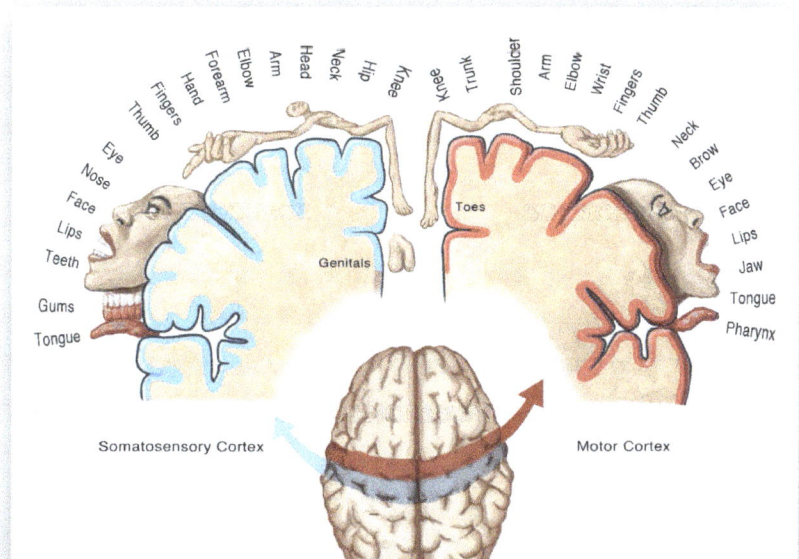

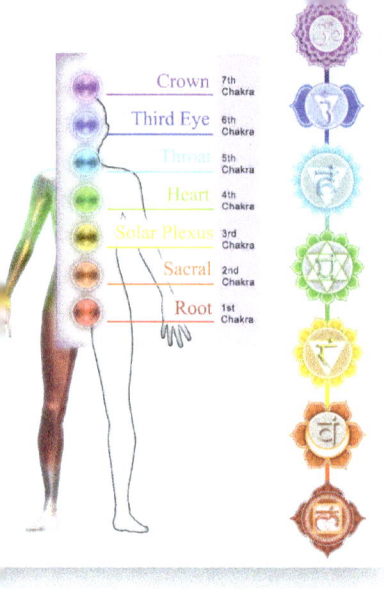

While enjoying a conversation, you can easily get absorbed into the details of the experience instead of resting in awareness; instead of being the calm center for your subtle bodies. When that happens, those experiences have to be processed like the food we eat, and how they are digested depends upon our personality's tendencies. Remember, it's not just your personality that's having the conversation; it's your entire being. If the exchange is harmonious on lofty subjects, or is brief and neutral, the reaction in the subtle fields and nervous system will be minimal, probably more balanced. A super fun, uproarious, or passionate conversation will create tons of stimulation.

It may then require a hot bath with sea salts and essential oils and a cup of chamomile tea to settle your system, but it may still reverberate in the night. Dreams are awesome ways to help process the day, and lucid dreaming, when you can show up consciously and affect the outcome, it helps even more. Nonetheless, you may attract an experience during the day that mirrors repressed subconscious layers. That's a good thing because the feelings generated are very helpful in bringing those impressions into awareness. The intelligence of the field will often create situations that accomplish this. It only works for your benefit if you recognize and claim the response as coming from old, stored impressions rather than blaming the situation or other person involved for your reaction.

One of those layers where subconscious memories are stored is in the nadis alongside the spine according to the Ancient Ayurvedic energy systems. Once the primordial life force—the kundalini energy at the base of the spine—becomes activated, as the Shakti rises up through these pathways, old memories and impressions will begin to surface. These in particular may not be initially recognized as to where they came from, but they will feel real to your senses, emotions, and energy. This energy can be triggered spontaneously, but meditation, shaktipat from a guru, or kundalini yoga can also set it in motion.

Feeling agitated afterwards could be a sign that these particles of the past are beginning to surface. They could create anxiety, depression, fatigue, tension, loss of sleep, digestive disturbances, headaches, and other side effects as they move from repressed energetic status to a state where you can sense them, but not be able to label them. There are books on the subject that cover what can happen if the kundalini energy begins to wake up and move. Just like with any other memory, remaining neutral to those stirrings permits them to be released harmlessly. Refining your ability to tune in to these areas alongside your spine, your heart, or

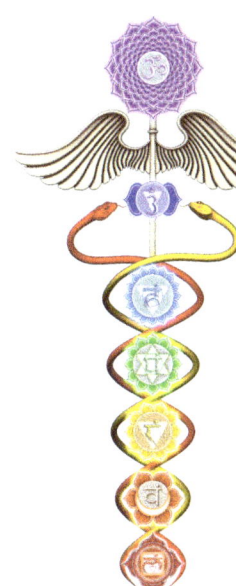

dan tien—that center beneath the navel—could prove a huge support in clearing those impressions, and freeing sources of knowing or wisdom. The right (Pingala) and left (Ida) channels spiral around the center (Sushumna) canal near your spine. As the Shakti clears restrictions from the other channels, it travels up the center canal on its way to the 7th chakra (Godhead) above the crown.

You will begin to feel aligned with those energetic bridges to deeper wisdom in your system that connect you with Spirit. In Ancient Chinese philosophy there are three dan tiens. One is two inches below the navel (2nd chakra), one is at the heart center (4th chakra), and one is between the eyebrows at the (6th chakra) third eye. In ancient Hindu philosophy, these are called chakras, or energy centers, where energy can be received, stored, and generated. Some use these centers as focal points for meditation. They also correspond in Western terms to the belly brain, heart brain, and brain/brain. They serve as antennae and bridges from the physical to the spiritual aspects of who we are. These centers will lead you into your deep body where freedom lives.

They can serve as major intersections where stored memories can safely exit the system and assume another, ideally, unconditioned form. The first law of thermodynamics states that energy cannot be created nor destroyed, it can only change form. The second law says that when energy changes from one form to another or moves freely in a closed system, disorder results. This is why so many spiritual practices or attempts to heal and evolve are filled with a bit of chaos. The Shakti releases restricted energy, life experiences attract and trigger subconscious patterns, and things will feel a bit shaky until it reorganizes into a more coherent form. Early on in the spiritual process this seems to happen a lot, but as time goes by, there just seems to be more equanimity in a broader range of situations because the triggers have been released.

Early stress or trauma can disconnect you from yourself and make you forget who you really are, and shroud some of those innate forms of knowing from being able to reach your conscious mind. Trauma orients you more toward the hind brain's fight/flight/freeze behavior instead of forward into the heart and prefrontal cortex. Self-sensing as the fulcrum and retaining the balanced baseline can reroute and reeducate the nervous system. It can also reprogram early and daily stressors. Meditating before going to bed is helpful, as is getting on the floor and doing a few movements to reorganize the soma in advance. The more your daily life content is released each day, the more likely it is that you can access your deep body.

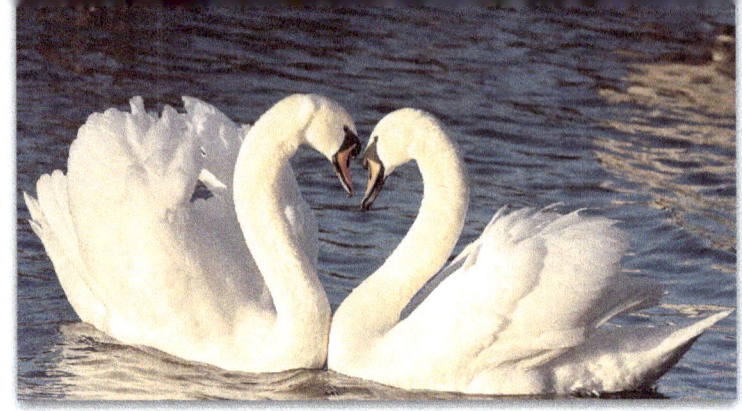

Our bodies respond to the harmonizing effects of the elements. For example, the water element is helpful in clearing and grounding some of the 'static' as it pours through the subtle fields in the shower. It also helps to wash away some of the extraneous particles. Using candles and tuning in to the radiance of the flame, or of the sun—the pure chi coming from the fire element—could do the same, especially for the eyes. Candles also helped clear the space at work and at home. Doing a practice under the night sky or on the earth were also ways of using the elements before bedtime to help return coherence within and in the subtle bodies.

Traditional medicine views illness or imbalance as a departure from those physical, energetic, and spiritual/natural laws, which are not separate from one another. They are also not separate from form. Full healing must include reconnecting these intricately woven forms of communication within their implicate order. David Bohm, a theoretical and mechanical physicist spoke at a conference in 1990 where he answered a question from a colleague, "…And if we have coherence, then what?" Bohm states, "We would produce the result we intend, rather than the result we did not intend. Then we would have more order, harmony and happiness. Unhappiness comes from incoherence."

## Pairing for electrical, energetic, and fluid flow

I began to notice something remarkable about pairing to open restrictions and creating more coherence. It was a technique we learned in Polarity Therapy using the natural electrical principles of the cell. You facilitate a movement of restricted charge by combing a positive with a negatively charged finger (thumbs are neutral) along a straight line. The line can be from front to back on a muscle, nerve, blood vessel, ligament or bone. It could be used along a horizontal, vertical, or diagonal using narrow or wide distances. The magnetic pull works on any combination of directions. I usually use the index finger of one hand combined with the middle finger or thumb of the other hand. Using the whole hand also works with right hand as positive and left hand as negative poles. I decided to use this method on my brain for the freezer bump symptoms. My left hand contacted the force outside of the side of my head, while my right hand touched a calm area of the brain.

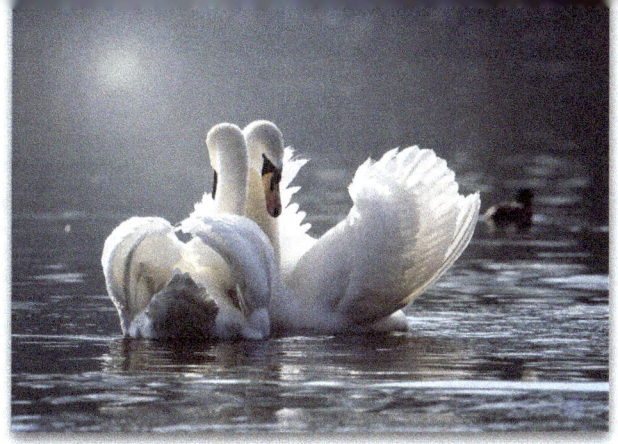

Pairing the noisy area in the field with a calm spot in the brain helped the agitation to recede by 75%. I moved the right hand a couple of times to other calm regions of my brain to see how the remaining 25% would respond. When I placed my right hand on the top, right part of my brain, a global response was elicited along the left side along with a bit of trembling as the shock took the form of a physical, energetic release. The force vector hand was now pulled into the right anterior cervical area and up into the supra-hyoid muscle under my chin (between the neck and the jawbone) which had been tight. Pairing this area with the hand following the force vector in the field was like the kingpin of the remaining 25%.

The sticky, stinging sensation in my neck had abated, along with 80% of the tinnitus-like sound that was now more like a tiny, high-pitched frequency that felt like it could be a section of the trigeminal nerve behind the ear. I worked with a few additional brain regions and membranes connected to the cranial nerves briefly, and another 20% reduction of 'buzz' followed. It confirmed my earlier experience that injuries need to be addressed on multiple levels for real healing to happen. It is also possible that you can access several layers within one system, if you adjust your attention and intention. It's a theory worth exploring.

After this, I was eager to explore that sticky area around the sternum using the pairing method. Working more thoroughly around the sternum, clavicle, and rib cartilage connections called up a response in the vascular structures underneath. This was surprising! The surface issue on fascia and bone had deeper roots. The tissue surrounding the chest and abdominal cavities as well the tissue (visceral peritoneum), surrounding all of the organs all joined in the conversation. The areas above the pulmonary arteries and veins were very sticky and heated, and releasing those areas brought immediate fulfillment to both lungs. A couple of ribs also needed adjusting, creating some of the same sensation of pressure and burning, along with the capture of the fascia.

Dr. Luigi Stecco, author and physical therapist, finds that overuse can create too much hyaluronic acid which under normal circumstances is a lubricant enabling fascial glide. Apparently, the increased amounts of this acid "aggregate into super-

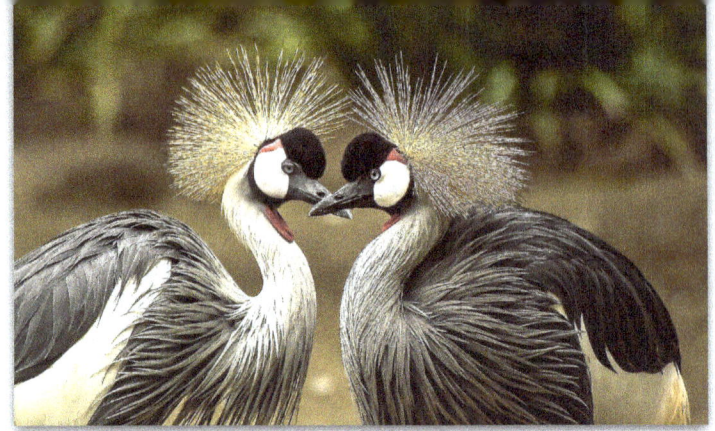

molecular structures changing both its configuration, viscosity, and viscoelasticity... which increases the resistance of the sliding layers and leads to densification of fascia, or abnormal sliding in muscle fibers." In my case it created this burning, sticky status that was a source of restriction, pain, and irritated nerve fibers.

However, opening these restrictions had wide-ranging effects. There was also gurgling all down through the belly, new releases through the thorax, kidney, and inguinal area, and unprecedented releases all the way down the spine and up into the sub-occipital region as though the vertebral artery had been primed like a pump. The freedoms gained through having this conversation with core vasculature also opened areas through the pelvis and thorax that I'd been seeking to release through breath and movement for decades. I imagine that the breath and prana, even meridian, and flow of energies had all been compromised by these restrictions. Prior to this exploration I couldn't sense the Conception vessel. After these releases, I could sense it, and the releases stayed unglued.

This Conception meridian is called the "Sea of Yin" or "Sea of Chi" and is connected to many organs as well as to the major energetic channels along the spine. Maybe those channels opened up and I thought it was the vertebral artery. Maybe they both opened up. Dr. Japa Khalsa says, "It is one of the most significant rivers in the body, carrying all yin fluids and making a loop with the Governing Vessel. The Conception and Governing Vessels are two of the 8 Extraordinary Meridians that act as tributaries to the 12 main meridians and share points with the organ meridians. The Extraordinary Meridians carry ancestral Qi and affect consciousness and the spiral of our genetic code. This is a direct parallel to the complexity of the Nadi system."

Considering that menopause often creates yin deficiency and excess of heat, that type of dehydration could be a place to look for support in resolving the sticky, burning effect in connective tissue that would be made even more intense with an injury. Wearing bras that constricted around the sternum and ribs added issues of discomfort in that area. For sure, the next exploration for me will be along the Governing vessel meridian, as its path straight up the midline in the back had

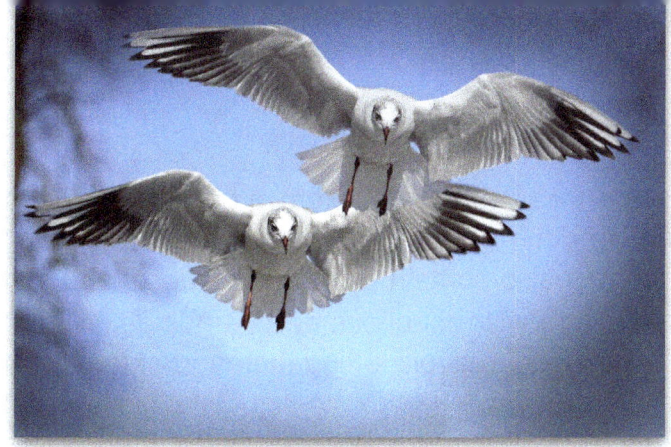

palpable tension. However, because I'm so flexible I can put my palms on the floor, my back didn't stand out as a place to look for a deeper integration. It's becoming clear that energetic systems are a source of necessary energy, repair, and nourishment that drive the healing process.

This process of addressing subtle sensations along with 'pulsing' paired spots with shared sensations created changes remarkably fast. I do believe that including the vascular system in the pairing mix will knock residual symptoms from recent injuries down to zero. You can get creative in the pairings. Consider matching part of the sensory cortex (shown on pg. 99) with a related body part. My favorite was the top of the head with my hip or thigh. You can try a meridian with an organ, a nerve with a muscle, a tendon with an artery, or anything that seems to share a sensation. They can be near to one another or at opposite ends of the body. They can be all in the physical arena, or you can pair an area of the subtle body with an area inside the physical form. Let your instincts and intuition guide you if not sensation. It can be any type of sensation. You begin by matching sensations of tenderness, sharpness, or whatever is most prevalent.

There's a distinct shift through the tissue when the polarities have recognized each other. If they're connected in a way that's significant, a therapeutic pulse will begin. In a few seconds, you will feel the tissue begin to open, lengthen, perhaps shed some heat and discharge. At that point, the area will feel like normal, healthy tissue again without any distinct sensation or tension attached to it. Create a movement using your arms and legs with the rest of your body afterwards to integrate the changes for the brain. Include wide, large movements along with more refined, smaller ones. The areas that take up the most space in the sensory-motor cortex (pg. 99) will be sending more input to your brain, so consider also creating small movements with your hands or with your mouth, tongue and lips.

I was astonished to see the global responses to making very tiny, conscious movements with my fingers and toes. It's well worth doing on a regular basis. The parts of our bodies that are in touch with the environment take in much more information every day, and could benefit a great deal from detailed reeducation. It's worth considering that these areas are often prone to arthritic changes, perhaps due to the fact that we don't think about releasing every joint on each finger and toe. Remember that they also contain entry and exit points to meridians as well as mini energy centers, along with countless nerve endings. When you think about it that way, it's more motivating to avoid letting them turn into storage facilities.

We, as awareness, can guide ourselves into, then beyond the senses we are most familiar with. When we do step out of that physical (food body) layer into clearing impressions in the subtle layers, real healing can happen. When we step past the clearing and healing in the subtle bodies into the deep body, we find wholeness. We discover our oneness with Existence as the Wisdom and Causal layer begin to reveal integration with the Whole where all things are possible. Feeling more deeply from within our connection to Mother Nature quite naturally develops into wonder, awe, and a more caring disposition towards her endlessly creative, life-giving, healing qualities.

## Finding your baseline and balance while standing

The 'finding baseline' exercise will be described next. The best outcome is that you'll discover your own unique holding patterns and how to unwind them. Make a mental note about the areas that are resistant to change and use them for pairing, or as a place to start to unwind future issues. We'll begin with some common associations that you can springboard from and modify according to what you find in your own body. For example, the hips and shoulders always work together, as do the arms and legs, like they do when an infant crawls. When you walk, if the right shoulder is forward, the right hip will be back. For that same reason, if there is holding in your shoulders, there will likely also be holding in the hips.

Let's see what you become aware of while we discover a resting tone as a baseline while standing. We will find where those snags in the fabric of your tissue fields might be that limit the effortlessness of that position in gravity. If you're not used to standing relatively still for several minutes, give yourself breaks and resume after working a little more with the area that's creating the most discomfort. For example, if your feet are responsible for the majority of the discomfort, you might not be able to make all of the necessary corrections needed while you're

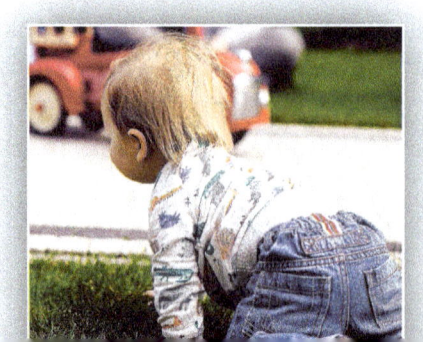

standing on them. It's fine to massage them, particularly in between the bones and down through your toes. Move them around to get residual tensions out so there isn't additional 'noise' in the system while you're trying to sense subtle changes.

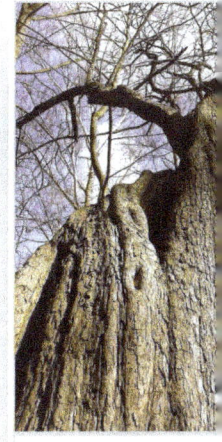

Initially, take a general scan and notice where your weight is. Is it more towards your toes or your heels; more on the right or left foot, or on the outer or inner sides of the feet? Then check to see if your pelvis is square or rotated, and do the same for your shoulders. Get a sense of whether your head and neck are forward, centered, or tilted, and of where your palms are facing. Bring your weight on your feet to neutral, then make tiny adjustments with your head and neck until they feel weightless on top of your spine.

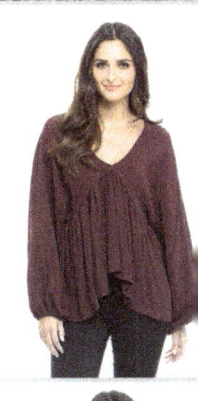

Now that we're reorganizing information from the upright posture, it will be easier to negotiate torsion if there is one. In the example with the women pictured to the right, you can see how a slight change in the position of the shoulders pivots the hips automatically and shifts where the arms and hands will lay. Bring your shoulders square on a straight horizontal line if you easily do so. If one shoulder was dropped and making one hand be lower on your leg, leveling your shoulders will fix that. The bottom image shows what happens to the skeleton if you drop your rib cage. Her upper back will be posterior, and her pelvis is jutting a bit forward. Can you tell if you've locked your knees and pushed your pelvis forward?

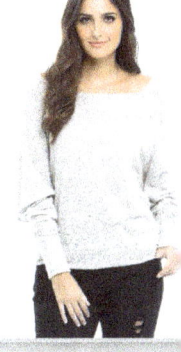

If so, bring it back so it feels like it's right under your neck and above your ankles, not in front of them. Over time it will create problems unless you catch it and level things out. Feel into those landmarks then recheck your system for sensations that grab your attention. Areas that are slightly out of alignment usually will create a little sensation. If self-sensing isn't giving you this information initially, you can look in a mirror. If a side-bend is present in the spine or pelvis, it will generally also add a slight rotation to counter-balance itself. Leveling your shoulders will correct the spiral and reveal if there's tension in your waist or in between your ribs. You'll feel it.

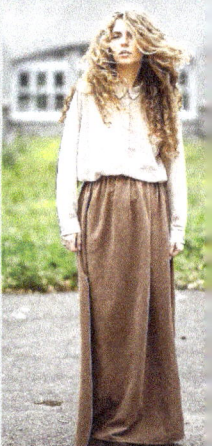

If there is, tilt your head to one side, wait a couple of seconds, then tilt to the other side and lift up again slowly. Notice which side of the neck pulls more down into your side. Repeat side-bending your neck, but this time rotate a little towards the ceiling. Your body will have released more of that tension for you when you come back to center. Check to see if you're twisting down through the legs or if it stops at the pelvis. Adjust the position of your feet until your hip joints and knees feel as comfortable and relaxed as they can.

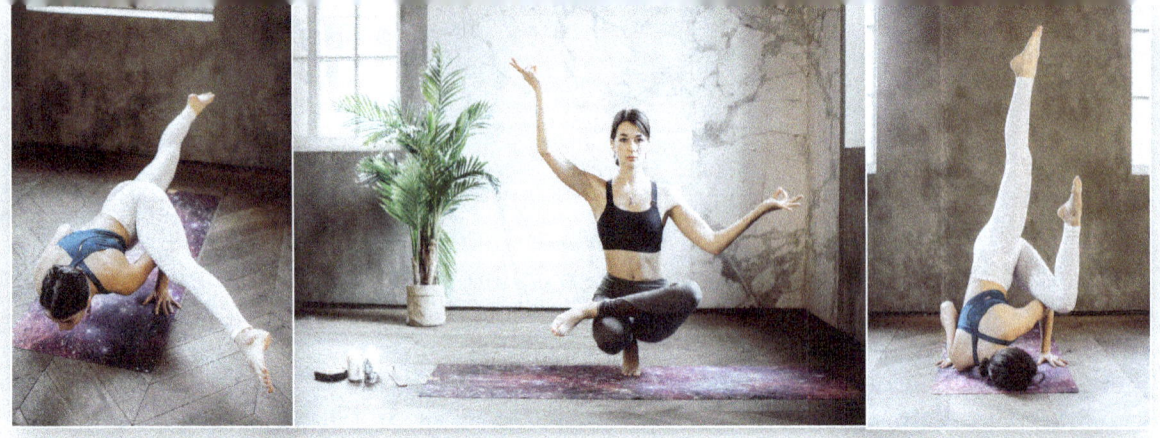

Be aware that walking around during the day with imbalanced forces on the feet and hip joints will also alter forces on the spine and knees. It's a good idea to do a quick 'diagnostic' for torsion before going out for a run or a long hike, if you're going to wear heels, or will be loading your structure with lifting during the day. Something as basic as constipation could be throwing things off in your center of gravity and create a mild internal shift, as well as the pelvic rotation pattern we spoke of earlier that can happen while driving. Try to remember the initial impetus your body may have had to shift out of alignment. That way you can keep track and notice if old scar tissue is responsible from a surgery, broken bone, or sprain.

We're looking for perfect symmetry, but we're aiming for optimal balance so that being in your body can feel effortless and pain-free. You want to be using only the muscular effort that is absolutely necessary to perform whatever function that is in front of you. That principle includes sitting or standing, because they are the basis for everything that happens next. So let's go a little farther now. Starting with the foundation you've already developed using the basic scan to release postural forces, make any additional mini-modifications that bring those loads into neutral. Lift and lower your shoulders a tiny bit a few times, move them forward and back a few times, take a few deep breaths and rest.

Alternate bending your knees a few times just a tiny bit, feeling what happens in your hips. Rock and rotate your pelvis in every direction slowly until the sensations diminish into a calm, neutral zone. Then tune into your spine in relation to your diaphragm and rib cage, which may be the epicenter of a spiral. Rotate your rib cage a tiny bit each direction, and feel for the direction of ease. See if you can move it while keeping your pelvis still. Lift your chest slightly and notice if there's more drag or resistance on one side. Let's call the side of resistance the direction of ease for side-bending. Side-bend a tad more in the preferred direction, then find the preferred direction for rotation and move slightly into that direction. Relax there, and find whether your body prefers to bend a little forward, or prefers to lean a little bit backwards. Follow that direction of preference/ease. Rest there, and your body will continue to unwind additional little areas of tension while you have them softened and in slack.

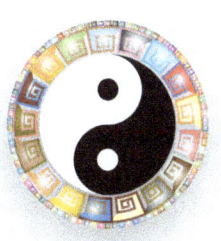
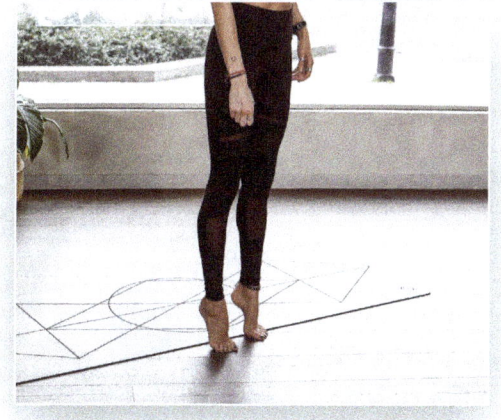
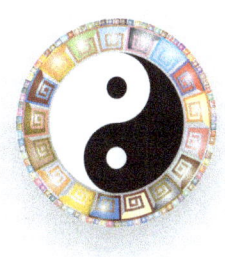

Breathe into it and wait for your body to stop making adjustments, then lift back up and recheck your overall ease of posture. Repeat on the other side, which will give you even more releases with minimal resistance. Experiment with adding a tiny bit more motion using a different angle; stacking another direction of ease, and pause at the end point chosen by your body. Return to neutral stance and tune in. Since we spend all of our time facing forward, your body may prefer to extend, it may fold in flexion, but take your body's suggestion whichever direction it leads you in.

Your system will learn to source its own internal restrictions and wind back out of them for you. If you're not being led yet, follow the planes of action—side bend, rotation, flexion or extension—and come back to center for the recheck. As a modification, you can explore turning your feet in or outward just an inch or two and repeat the exercise. In each new position of ease, as well as when coming out of it, go slowly, allowing your brain to assess and record the changes. Then lift up onto your toes and rest there for a couple of seconds, followed by lifting your toes and feet so that you're resting on your heels. Use a soft enough surface so that it's comfortable, but not so soft as to not afford stability for balance.

This will stimulate many regions of your brain as it tries to accomplish the balance on such a small area of your feet, but this stimulation will awaken more receptors in both areas and improve it, along with your posture. Focus attention on your rib cage and thorax while your awareness remains global. Take a deep breath and notice if any area stands out as feeling more restricted to a full breath than the rest. Notice if that area tends to create a slight pull of your rib cage in any direction. Next, take a deep breath, hold it in, and gently place soft fists on the sides of your ribs int the R 3-8 area. The body will begin to make many subtle adjustments as the internal membranes around the lungs are given a bit of slack.

Release your pressure and exhale as those adjustments come to conclusion. Take a deep breath, exhale and hold it, and repeat the above, now using a different osmotic pressure in the chest cavity. If there begins a slight motion or downwards by your body, gently follow and enhance the opening with your hand, but just with an ounce of pressure. Repeat the same with both the inhale and exhale while turning your toes in just a couple of inches to open the sacroiliac joint slightly.

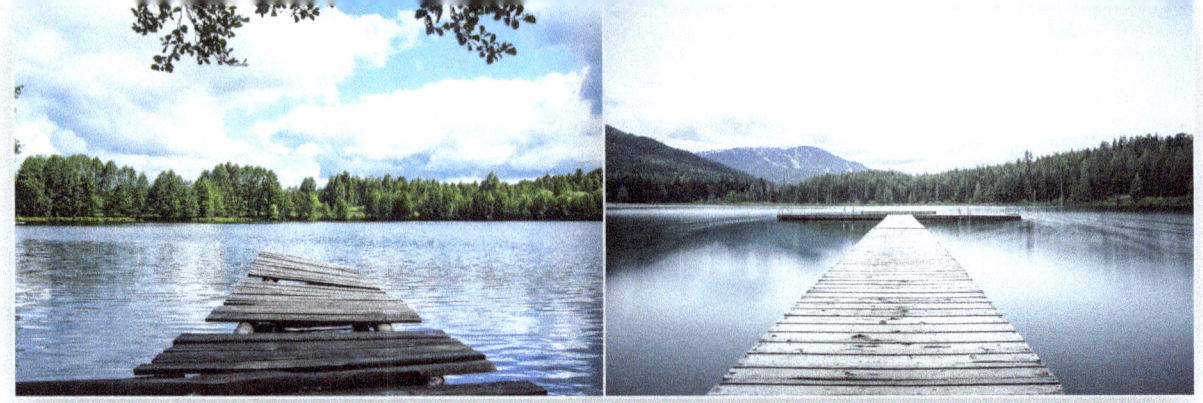

Come back to your baseline resting tone with global awareness and take a few deep breaths to inform the brain of the new openings. Although you and your body are communicating throughout these explorations, and your awareness is present while the changes are happening, it's still helpful for your body and brain to retain the information exchanged by using a movement that reinforces the fact that there are new freedoms present.

You've created positional and postural updates that the brain needs to integrate. Do that now. Create some wide, stretching movements with your whole body, then come back to relaxed, balanced, posture. If you can get your hands up higher under your armpits to do a compression up there to repeat the exercise, it would be very beneficial. The upper ribs become easily compressed due to the weight of our shoulders and the things we lift and carry during the day. You may want to loosen your fingers so that they're flat instead of curled into a fist for this to feel less awkward. Be gentle and slow going in, and appreciate that sensitive, listening organs are underneath the areas you're applying pressure to.

## Organizing the core

Another area that is ripe for receiving the reorganizing of your posture in any position is the spinal cord at the core of your body; the midline. A torsion in bony connections or membranes inside the skull or in the vertebrae of the spine could generate subtle forces that would cause soft tissue to shift in many areas of your body, starting from the midline outward. Now that many significant peripheral issues have been resolved, the core tensions will be easier both to identify and to balance. If you're not in the cranial field, or aren't in a manual therapy practice that is familiar with how to address these (sphenoid, dura, tentorium, faux, vertebral body) structures, you may need to have a practitioner sort that out for you. Subtle, specific movement practices may be able to reach some of them by reorganizing the spine, adjacent muscles, and fascia that run all the way up to the head. There are many movement sequences that work the tiny muscles along the spine in concert with the legs, neck, and head that could provide amazing results with this.

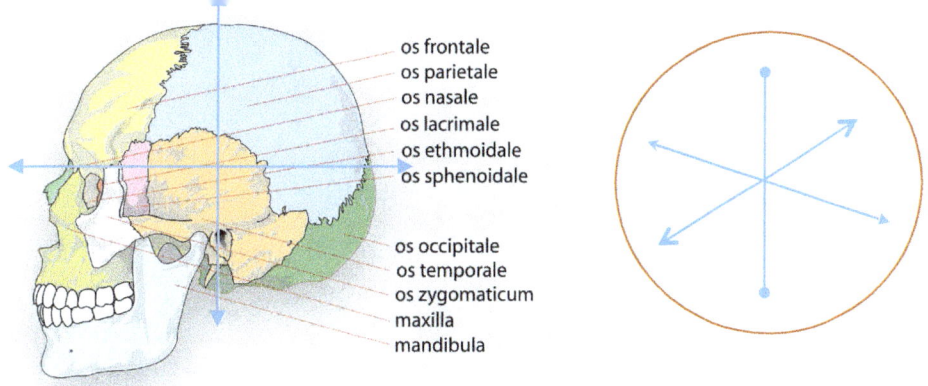

If you are a manual therapist with cranial/brain familiarity, you can check for bony alignments as well as resting your hands on the top of your head above the coronal suture and feel for any restrictions in motion or any rotational forces upon the brain. Giving the brain a frame of reference is immensely helpful for it to be able to re-orient itself in space. Envision a beam of light, or a straight line down through the crown from the position above and slightly behind the mastoid bone, so that the line carries into the spine. The imaginary line will give the brain an axis to organize around and help it to be seated squarely in the midline.

I sometimes pick a central point that a line could intersect from each plane—transverse, coronal, and sagittal—and envision a line extending out in each direction. This would be the image of a three-dimensional cross, perhaps at a slight posterior angle to follow the line of the 4th ventricle. Further study of the Primo Vascular System found a fiber of this system running through the fourth ventricle. Therefore, that may also be a significant place to add some attention, if not a line of intention. The brain, and in fact any juncture in the body, will recognize these trajectories and will use them as a point of reorganization.

These directional visualizations can also be used in the joints, through an individual vertebra, or through energy centers. I also use them through the sternum, and out through the shoulders and the heart, and through the vascular exchange through the lungs, and at the center of gravity (dan tien) while holding the superior to inferior pole down the spine. It's particularly wonderful to use it going through third ventricle since it's such a hub of activity and is in line with the straight sinus and Sutherland's fulcrum. It is best to use this at the end of all other methods of balancing and settling the system, as it is one of the more subtle methods that may otherwise yield its influence to stronger forces.

Dr. Barral says, "The body hugs the lesion." For example, if you've had a recent injury or one that hasn't fully healed, it may express as a pull towards the issue. If you touch your body lightly with your hand, the force will literally move your hand. That pull could manifest as a rotation, side-bend, tissue distortions or a leaning towards an area that needs attention. This force may represent an adhesion that will overpower any visual suggestion. If there is a correction that is resisting the return to midline, it's better to follow the pull, and address it first. In general, it's

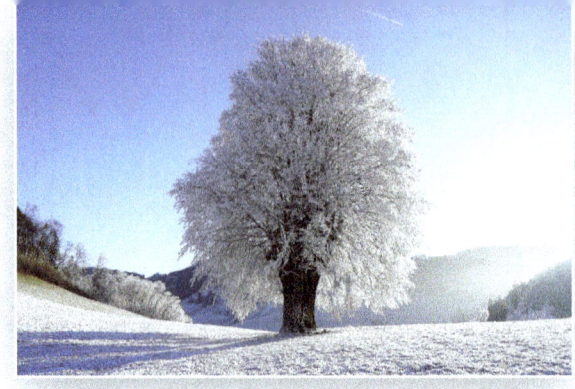

more effective to first release the stronger forces at play. Once released, the system will automatically orient itself towards midline; towards a more neutral status. Then the more subtle and smaller structures can be informed by the subtle (i.e. visualization) input suggestions without distraction.

If there's a large, or deep scar, it's more likely that you'll just have to check it from time to time, or remember those signals from the body that tell you when to use your method of releasing it. There are many essential oils that can be used to help prevent scarring, but deep scars from surgeries or C-sections will need treatments like cross-fiber or myofascial techniques to periodically unwind those thickened, grabbing tissues. It could seem like a small scar from a laparoscopic surgery but if it happens to be in a complex, intricate area like the foot, neck, pelvic bowl, knee or the groin, a constant pull on a ligament, vessel or nerve could have a major impact.

There are warm compresses or oils that penetrate more deeply into the skin and have impressive amounts of nutrients, emollients, essential fatty acids, anti-oxidants, and more. Applying them will soften the adhesions and reduce the extent of the grab in the scar tissue, but most likely the pattern will be something that needs ongoing monitoring. It may be one of the places to look first when an imbalance arises. The adhesions from the sprains in my ankles made the area more vulnerable to irritation decades later, and also were responsible for my system having difficulty orienting itself in space accurately.

During the rolling ball incident that rang my brain's bell, a patch of eczema that was healing on that ankle got beet red and painfully sensitive as if the skin had been burned. It had never been like that before. It was never more obvious that the central nervous system was connected to the peripheral and subcutaneous systems and this top-down injury through the midline was a scorcher that echoed out through several systems. Because of the adhesions in that foot and ankle, the blood flow in and out was restricted, the immune function in the tissue field and skin was reduced, and the nerve signaling was impaired.

I did, by the way, use yogurt with probiotics inside to apply to that patch of eczema after I learned that the skin had its own microbiome. Just like the brain injury, this injury of the skin had to be treated on several layers. I approached it through anti-

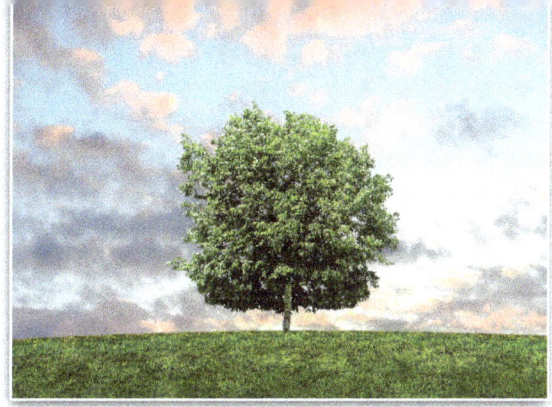

inflammatory creams and antiseptic oils, fatty acid balancing oils, oils to protect and mend the nervous system, oils to stimulate the production of new skin cells and reduce scarring, and nourishing oils. I also used extracts with vitamins, minerals, amino acids, herbal salves to reduce scarring, to break up the adhesions, along with steroidal creams. I tried opening energy flow through the meridians, decompressing the bones, and more. Even with all of this, the rash wasn't responding much until the main aspects of the brain injury were out of the woods.

I'd like to emphasize again what a unique creature a brain injury is. For as multi-faceted as any injury proves to be, when the brain becomes faulty, the healing process becomes even more tenuous and unpredictable. The stages and systems that it fluctuates through may set up an erratic way of responding that you have to navigate with patience, and a willingness to knock on a different door when the musculoskeletal system is in a holding pattern. It may release, but then snap back again a few times. Many of the same principles of finding a baseline for neutral balance, contrast and noise reduction still apply. However, due to phases of inflammatory processes and of inaccurate signaling, some of the vocabulary you'd normally use to create changes may not work in the normal, more lasting ways.

These systems will now have unspecified routes of reorganization as the nerve cells gradually come back on board, or are replaced so they can use the familiar vocabulary again. In addition, the fluid systems, energetic pathways, viscera, biochemical pathways, and other doors you could usually communicate through will also be under a readjustment process. Volume 6 goes into great detail as to the many modalities that can be used to help bring all the affected systems back up to speed, but here it will suffice to say that it takes more time than other types of injuries. The brain, more than others, will tend to seek global, comprehensive solutions. Nonetheless, and even more so in these instances, orienting down through the midline and using the three-dimensional cross inside the brain and down the spine is a tremendous way to assist in the reeducation process.

In that same area of the midline along the central channels as well as in the heart there is a stillness. There is a very, very quiet zone that was mentioned earlier as one of the most helpful ways to support and reorient the brain and central nervous

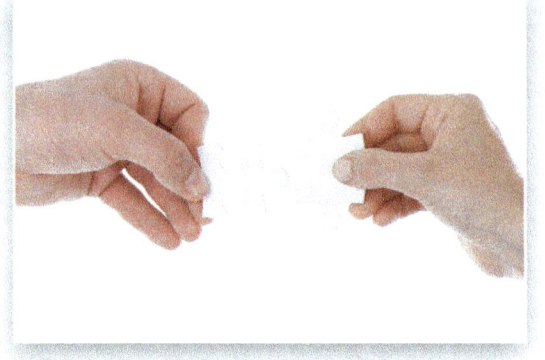

system. Listening to that sound deep to the ear drums rather than tuning outward towards external sounds is almost as beneficial as deep sleep. One of my teachers called it, "The sound of one hand clapping". Similar to the effect of pulling the attention behind the eyes, pulling the attention to listen inward is super soothing for the cranial nerves, as well as for the brain and the descending pathways.

## Pairing key locations as context for the brain

Using the pairing explorations described earlier can deepen somatic integration while revealing which different systems are involved in the pattern. For example, you may be using a movement that reveals tension along your ribs, then as you continue the motion it becomes obvious that the (IT) iliotibial band and same side of the neck are also tight. This is a pretty common combination ,and conscious motion is usually effective way to increase freedom in all of these areas. However, if you're tuning into your muscles and one of the restrictions is in the vascular system, the release won't be complete and the freedom/integration will be limited.

In addition, ischemic (tight, oxygen-deprived) tissue fields relax and open to a greater information exchange, as well as glide when nerves and vessels are free. If there is an ongoing soft barrier while moving, it's best to check other systems to see where the 'hang up' is, and proceed again. You can use the pairing technique on blood vessels and nerves; it works beautifully there. As we move into the pairing exploration, see whether you notice a little area being less fluid or less free, even though it can continue the movement without pain. If the snag remains during very gentle, slow movement and you know there isn't, for example, osteoarthritis (hard barrier) in that joint responsible for the restriction, check the neighboring major artery. We can do a brief, general check now.

If while standing or moving you discover tension in your hips that keeps coming back no matter what you've tried, it may be the common/internal/external iliac, or femoral arteries. Ever so gently place a finger or two above the inguinal ligament at the junction between your belly and your thigh. Feel for the pulsing of the femoral artery and wait for a shift in the tissue. It usually begins to soften the area right away. Arteries are easy to find because they pulse with the same rhythm as the heart. It may guide you to a restriction adjacent to the artery. Make contact at the

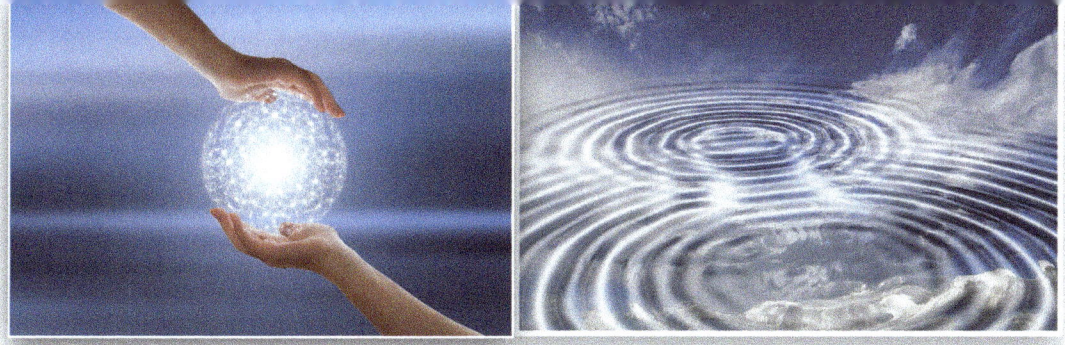

ligament and notice if there's a pull up into the abdominal area, out into the hip area, or down into the thigh. Make the second contact if you feel the pull to do so.

Apply gentle pressure above the artery that's under the ligament, and listen for an echo in another area along its path. If you're not sure, put the next finger below your navel for spot number 2. Wait a couple of seconds and allow the tissue to unwind in response. Then notice which section of the artery feels more full compared to the 'quieter' sense of flow. Gently connect them and wait for them to pulse together in recognition. Once they begin to pulse, pull back the light pressure and wait for them to complete their 'conversation'. When the reduced flow area has a stronger pulse and the tissue field responds by opening and softening, remove your hands. Then initiate gentle movement and track the changes in soft tissue.

Of course, if you feel any hesitancy in treating your own arteries, just make a mental note and see an osteopath first before trying it yourself. They are not fragile structures and enjoy being stretched, but not compressed. It's helpful to realize that there may be another layer of your system that is influencing the soft tissue, and ischemia is something that doesn't always respond to stretching, movement, or massage. This is more specific and will be able to resolve the issue if it's caused by vessels near the surface. Otherwise pulsed magnetic frequency devices are able to access capillaries and deeper structures.

Return to your balanced standing baseline and rest in neutral. Notice any increase of ease in your hips and arms. Step out to the side with your right foot, and find a balanced stance with your weight evenly distributed between both feet. Notice which area is producing more sensation in that position. From here, slightly bend one knee, then the other, and notice the effect in your pelvic and hip areas. Repeat the motion and sense what is happening in your shoulders during this bending of the knees. Keep going and make small circles with your shoulders as you move, letting that motion as well as the one with your hips be a smooth as it can be. Once you've smoothed it out, slow each motion down and see if you can still maintain the smoothness.

Come back to neutral stance and sense what may have changed during the movement. Let those changes register, and pause a few seconds to see if your body will continue making adjustments, or point out any other restriction. Begin the

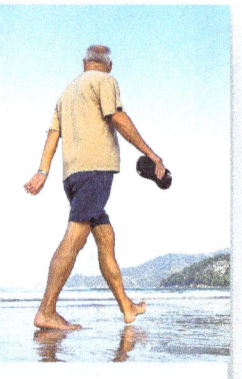

motion again, this time varying the position of your hands. Start with the palms facing your thighs, then rotate your arms and shoulder joints externally so that your palms are facing forward. Maintain soft wrists and elbows, letting them bend if it feels natural for them to do so. Repeat one more time with your palms facing behind you, keeping the motion as smooth as you can. You may find that you're reorganizing and balancing patterns used in walking. Imagine yourself carefree and in your favorite place as you move and let that felt-sense flow through you.

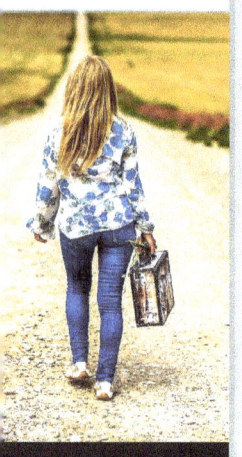

Rediscover your neutral baseline, and allow for slight adjustments your body may offer as it continues to receive feedback about the recent input. From that balanced stance, keep your arms still by your sides while you make circles with your pelvis and thorax. Find whichever way feels the most graceful and natural, as you slightly lift your shoulders one at a time to allow more space for the core to move freely. Smooth it out and slow it down, gliding as effortlessly as you can. Tune into your inner dancer and hear your inner music as though you were moving under water, and see if your body creates different movements using those descriptives. Move again, this time including your arms and varying your hand positions.

Now that you feel balanced in stasis and in motion, close your eyes while in resting baseline stance and scan your internal sense to see if your felt sense in the outer soma matches the felt sense inside. Do you notice any pulls and torques with your inner eyes that you didn't notice with eyes open? If so, take a deep breath and hold it while you place a vertical line down through the core from crown to perineum. Wait for the body to make adjustments. Then open your eyes and look up; straight up towards the center of your eyebrows. Notice if there is a slight pull to the left or to the right, and if there is ease or tension in one eye more than the other.

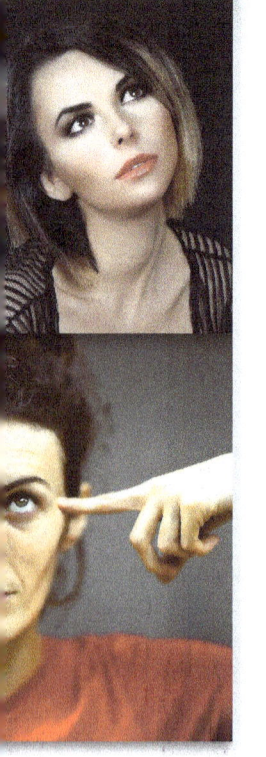

If you do notice a pull, place a finger lightly on your temples and see if there is also a slight pull there. You may feel at this juncture of the sphenoid a little rocking back and forth, and as long as it continues to rock evenly it's fine. If the position of this junction feels slightly off balance, keep a finger next to the eye socket, and place one finger of each hand on your cheekbone, and another on the edge of your eyebrows and wait for your eyes to respond. Lift your chest, hold your belly in, and wait again for another set of adjustments. Tilt your head at different angles while moving your eyes up, down, left, and right and at angles high and low. Be aware of tensions in any direction while your fingers are at the eye orbits.

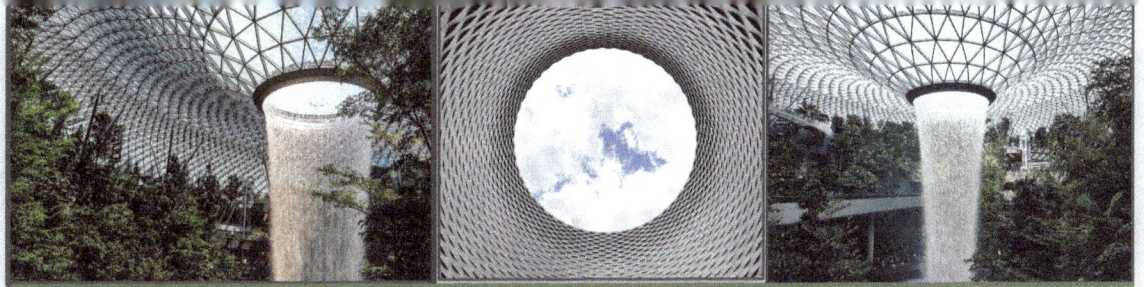

We are almost always looking straight ahead or down, so the tension will most likely appear when you look up at an angle, the direction least in use by us. Once you've discovered the position with the most tension while your fingers are lightly placed, gently move your pelvis, then your shoulders in small circles. Come back to center and wait for your brain to process the input and make the adjustments. Now recheck the freedom in the movement of your eyes. Since the eyes are connected to everything we do, it's helpful from time to time to free them from their pairing with other motor patterns that they've been temporarily wired within.

Now that your body, your system, and your eyes are freer and more balanced, more in tune, in touch, and integrated throughout, take a moment to sense what is looking out through your eyes and expressing through your body. What is the disposition, the energetic quality or characteristic, the state of you as the fulcrum and superior officer? Take a moment and try on a few adjectives for yourself with your eyes closed. Notice what changes in your face and energy when you label yourself as 'happy,' 'peaceful,' 'energized,' 'young,' 'fresh,' 'tired,' 'weak,' 'strong,' 'supple,' 'awesome'. Feel the ways in which your cells mold themselves to mirror your perceptions of yourself. Think over which words your body was the most responsive to that you may now use as a frame of reference for what you want to inspire in your nervous system.

Hear, feel, and see that your entire system listens, responds, and adapts to you as the organizing principle that it is in sync with. Explore other imaginings or archetypes you'd like to in-form your system with to see which resonates the most as being aligned with what you see your being moving into. It's fun sometimes to put an image of your face when you were younger into your current face and watch the molecules of your tissue field begin to shift in accord. If you look in an actual mirror, your current face will reflect those changes, as well as with some of the other dispositions you begin to embody. If there are physical issues you'd like to see and feel differently, envision that also and listen to your system as it responds.

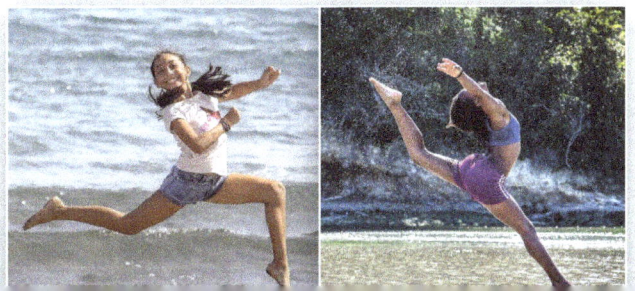

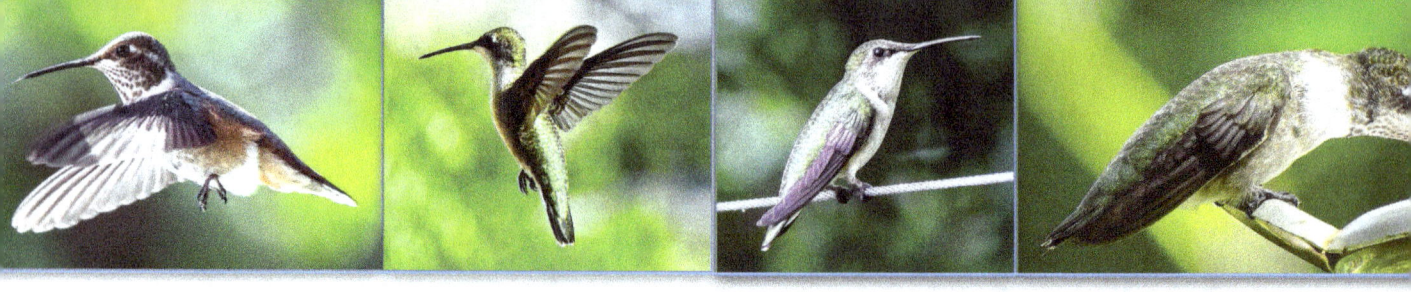

## Creating cellular space

There are delicate, exquisitely sensitive sensors in your body that respond to the slightest input. Think in terms of the weight of a feather, or a baby chick's fur, or a motion that is the distance of the width of a hair. Our bodies can detect and reply to these tiniest increments of input in a host of ways that result in changes according to your intention and its own knowing. It does help to be quiet inside neurologically, physically, and mentally so that these smallest of cellular exchanges can be perceived. It may help to be sitting down in this exploration so the muscles that keep you upright can be relaxed. We will be sensing the space in between fibers, in between cells, and into flows of energy, as tiny particles of information become active within the silent field within.

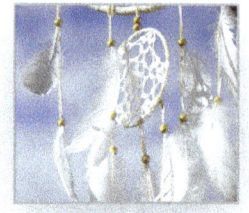

Dr. R. Paul Lee quotes Newman and Tomasek's (1996) observation that, "Cells recognize and respond to mechanical stresses by changing their shape, growth, expression of specific gene products, and cytoskeletal organization, as well as by remodeling their extracellular matrix within minutes of perturbation." It may take longer than that for these changes to manifest in what we'd notice as a symptom, but it could be helpful to view this molecular level of activity as a place we can possibly influence and help balance. This study shows the result of even tiny changes: "When mechanical stressors are removed from cells, cAMP production, arachidonic acid levels, and intracellular calcium levels increase, all consistent with the healthy functioning of the cell." (He Y and Grinnel F, *J of Cell Biology* 1994)

Remember that feeling of spacious weightlessness that happens after having released internal forces? Could you sense that as a result being integrated and aligned with gravitational forces? Tune into that space again from the resting baseline. Your awareness is global around and within your system, engaged lightly with no particular focus. Once you're there, allow your attention to be drawn into the local spot or zone that is vibrating more than the rest; that's sending more sensation. Realize that some restrictions are related to a very minuscule section of a nerve, or lining of a vessel, or strand of connective tissue, that a large motion will miss. That said, search for the tiniest of restrictions.

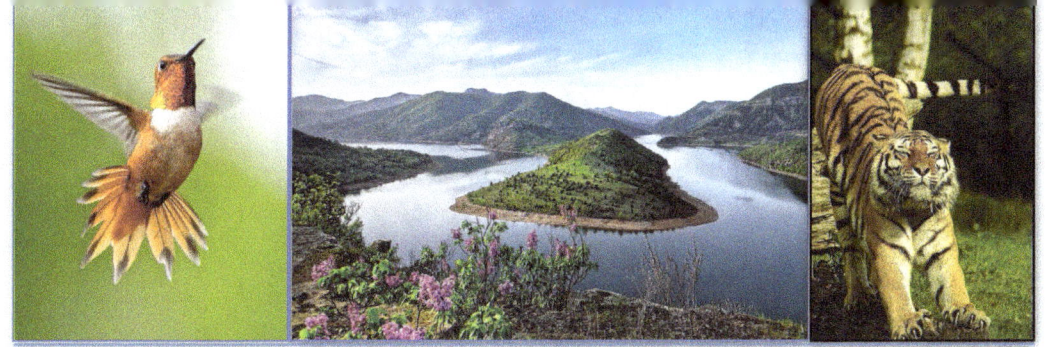

Here we will tune into the slightest of sensations and listen for an echo in another area. It might the brain, the spine, an extremity, a bone; remain open to it being anywhere. When you find the first spot, move it just one millimeter either in rotation or side-bending and wait for the response somewhere else. After you've identified the second spot, initiate a very tiny motion that connects them. It may be a global movement though you're specifically dialed into a very, very tiny area, moving one spot towards the other, then away from each other. The movement is about the width of a hair in both directions. Be inside of the first spot with your presence and pause when the motion is complete. After your system responds again, enter the echoing area with your presence. While you're there, see if any other area lights up as part of the pattern.

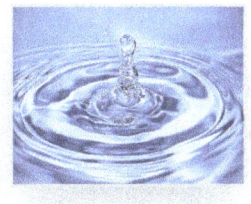

It could be your belly, a foot, a meridian, the thymus, a thought process; any source of input from an area that may be vibrating into and sharing the pattern. If there is, embrace them all with your presence enter into the vibration/sensation by finding a miniscule space inside of it. You want to enter not what is solid there, but go in between the fibers, in between the cells; find the spaces behind or between. You can also try sensing the fluid inside of, or between the sensations the tiny structure is producing. After these subtle changes have registered in your system, feel into the vibrating regions again and make note of what's left, if anything. Now you can experiment with making the slightest change in the position of a joint that is closest to one of the areas in the pattern.

Continue in this process of altering joint positions in your ankles, knees, shoulders, elbows, wrists, as they call to you, or as you sense a tiny activation that is connected to the pattern. Move your eyes in different directions and monitor which direction increases holding of the pattern, and which directions support the release and softening of the holding or vibration. There may be a spot where a release begins to happen from the system based upon that pairing with the eyes. Wait there for the discharge to complete, then move in a smooth pattern until there's another soft barrier with your eyes. Continue the process until your eyes and joints feel as free as they can with this particular exercise, then return to baseline and settle in.

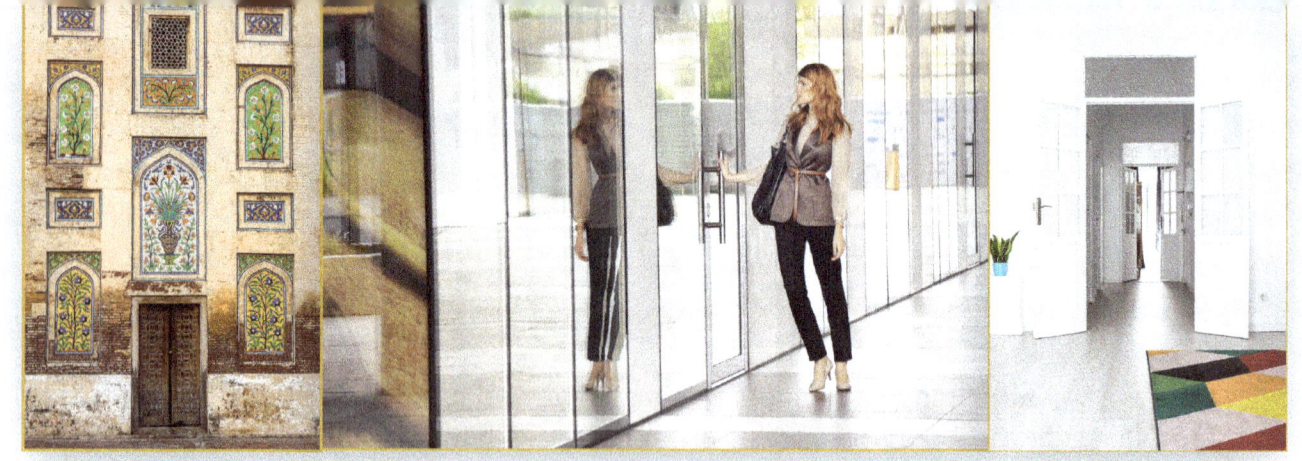

## Opening space in the core

We've released the extremities, so now it's time to move into the core and create space there. Begin at the tailbone and sense the four very small sections of the coccyx (your tailbone). This may be a sticky area if you've fallen on it or have broken it in the past. If you've lost sensation in this area, move laterally onto the small muscles between the coccyx and the ischial tuberosities (sit bones) of the pelvis, or on the adjacent (sacrococcygeal or sacrotuberous) ligaments. Don't worry if the two sides of your body feel different from one another; there may be different reasons. For many traditions the left side represents the feminine, receptive side, while the right is the masculine, expressive side. The energies may be manifesting differently, or you may have been using your dominant side differently throughout your life.

These could be subtle influences worth exploring. The difference may also be coming from the brain. In any case, they may not feel the same from one day to the next, as many things determine how energies and tensions manifest. Let's explore and see what turns up. Sense up into the most inferior landmark of your sacrum with your awareness and work your way up. Pay attention to which area begins to release the unilateral tension pattern if one side sticks out more than the other. See how small your presence can be made in each area as if you can easily penetrate the cells within; not piercing them, more like a soft breeze entering.

If it feels more like tenderness or soreness rather than stiffness, make a mental note without trying to make them feel identical. Check it again in other activities to see if you can identify anything that may be contributing to the tenderness. Once you know, use the baseline balance method to find a neutral posture for that activity. Now, come up to the apex of the sacrum, the joint where it meets the base of the spine. In these areas, you may notice a slower response time than in a tissue field. It could take several seconds for the joint space to begin to notice itself and send down a change. It may feel like the speed of a row boat, a sailboat, a

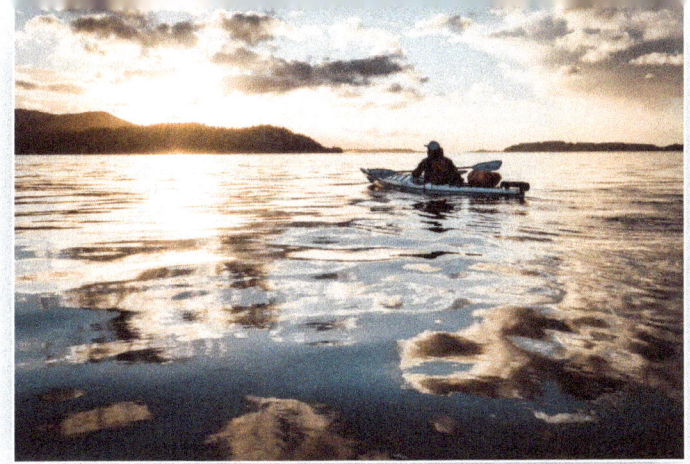

kayak, or a cruise ship. However it is for you, once you feel like the area has awakened enough so that it's sending back a sensation to your awareness, let your presence penetrate the joint and pour between the cells that make up the cartilage there. Then just wait for the 3-D changes to begin and complete their gradual adjustments.

You can tell that the brain has recognized the area that your presence is pointing out when you feel slight adjustments begin to happen on their own. New sensations will fill the area as the lights become turned on and space enters. Be patient with those intricate, intimate niches that you're knocking lightly on the door of, as they will come to answer in the safe space that you create for them. You can also keep track of what happens in this area during the arch and curl movement, or within other integrating explorations that may reveal which area is related to the restriction. Consciously pulse and pair them once you find out.

As we visit the core of our bodies, which can also be considered as the core of our beings, there may be memories that come from ancestral lineages or even from your soul's experience at another time and place. If they do and you don't recognize what may arise in an image or feeling, there is no need to claim anything, but just to acknowledge it and let it pass through. Who knows which way the iconic parts of our brains and memories may have attached to experiences and recorded them? It may very well be abstract or symbolic like a dream, but somehow meaningful to parts of you at the time they became stored there. They could also show up being vivid and specific in a flash that you don't recognize, or as a section of a forgotten story being unearthed in fuzzy, but familiar context.

Sometimes, the deeper memories are in the bones and in the tinier places that can easily be overridden in a busy life, even within spiritual practices or gentler movement practices. The readiness is in the intelligence of the system, the readiness versus any attachment by you as the fulcrum, and the quality of the trust and safety therein. The body is never judging the situation from a critical point of view, and it's helpful if you, as the fulcrum, also let the circumstances associated with it remain free as well.

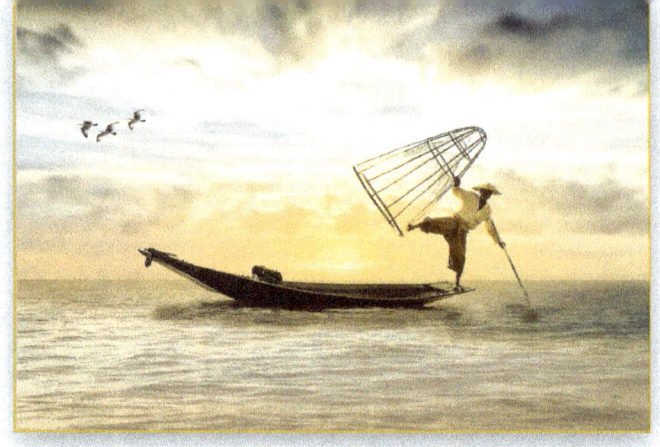

It may be stitched in with a variety of other experiences in amazingly creative ways that can be surprisingly elegant and clever if you look inside the storyline of how the body processed it. Just remember that your system is always doing its best to work with you in the most caring and effective way possible. Early in my spiritual process there were many images and memories that didn't seem to belong to me, but yet evoked a powerful response from my body. Each time afforded new freedoms internally after letting the images have a voice, and acknowledging how they were interpreted by my system. These types of hidden, mysterious stories can produce somatic symptoms whiccan be sorted out with self-sensing and by having regular conversations with your body to help decode and guide the feedback in a clearer direction. Sometimes free-flow journaling with your non-dominant hand can also produce revelations.

So take your time sensing up your spine, and follow your instincts or your body's signals when to take a break. Explore pairing each segment of the spine with any other area of sensation that may light up at the same time and let them connect. Hold them in your awareness until you feel the connection happen. Fan out laterally a bit at each juncture to include the small muscles adjacent to the vertebrae. Compare each side and make tiny adjustments in articulations until you feel a balancing happen. Come deeper with your awareness toward the spinal cord in front of the vertebral arch and behind the vertebral body, and notice any tendencies toward shortening or rotation on one side versus the other. If there is a rotational shift happening, hold your intestines securely and squarely and sense again.

While holding them, arch and curl slightly and notice again if there are restrictions in movement more on one side versus the other. Bend your knees as you curl. If there is, press more deeply in toward the iliopsoas and recheck. Do what you know to do to balance tone in the iliopsoas region and place your hands opposite one another around the bottom of the ribs with your attention on the diaphragm. Give it a moment for your system to make its own internal adjustments under your hands as there are several structures attached to, and passing through the center of this area. Inhale and exhale a couple of times to see how the attachments of the

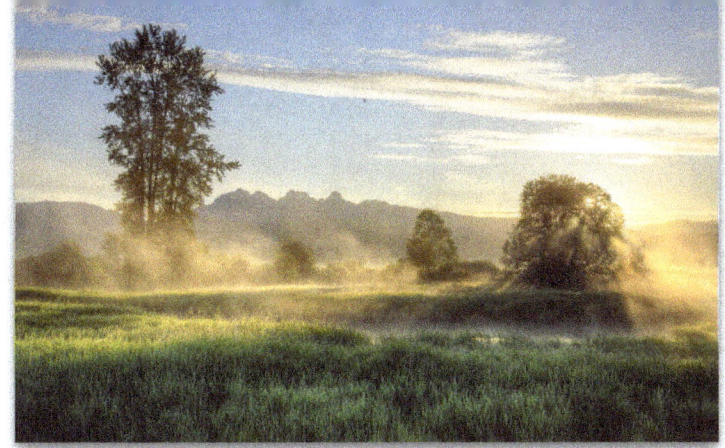

diaphragm respond. Inhale and feel what changes in your belly as the diaphragm shifts downwards, and feel what happens again as you exhale. Repeat with your toes turned in, and once again with them turned out, feeling which position brings more thoracic ease.

Are there any global changes throughout your posture now? Let's return to light arches and curls with your low back, then continue through the whole spine as you cradle the rib cage and diaphragm with your hands. Make note of where the ease or tensions are as you slide your attention up the cord all the way to the base of the skull. Flex your head and neck as you reach that level of the spine. Modify the action by making your breath as quiet and smooth as possible, and move your thumbs posterior on the ribs just enough to have a sense of the adjacent ligaments supporting the liver and spleen. Compress just a tiny bit there as you begin the motion again, being aware of the glide or stickiness you may feel along the way in the tissue fields just beneath your ribs.

If the ribs feel a little tender, glide them just a hair in towards and away from your spine with your thumbs. Next time through the movement, shift your hands to your pelvis, press in slightly during extension, and release during flexion. While maintaining global awareness with local attention on the core, pay attention to the nerve fibers connecting the spinal cord to the tailbone. Knowing where they are now, the filum terminale and cauda aquina, as you flex the spine, does one side move more easily than the other? Sense the connection between these fibers under the sacrum down to the coccyx, and where they begin around L1/L2.

Is there more of a tug on one side than the other? Are you able to do a smooth flexion, or does it wiggle slightly side-to-side? If so, squeeze your pelvis slightly as you move it around gently in a few directions, then come back and check if flexion is any easier. Be sure to lift your head and entire spine towards the ceiling and stretch your tailbone away from the spine as you arch. Move laterally just a tad with your attention that's tuned in to the cord just onto the denticulate ligaments that attach to and support the meninges. Side bend slightly to sense them more clearly and test for glide or stickiness at each segment.

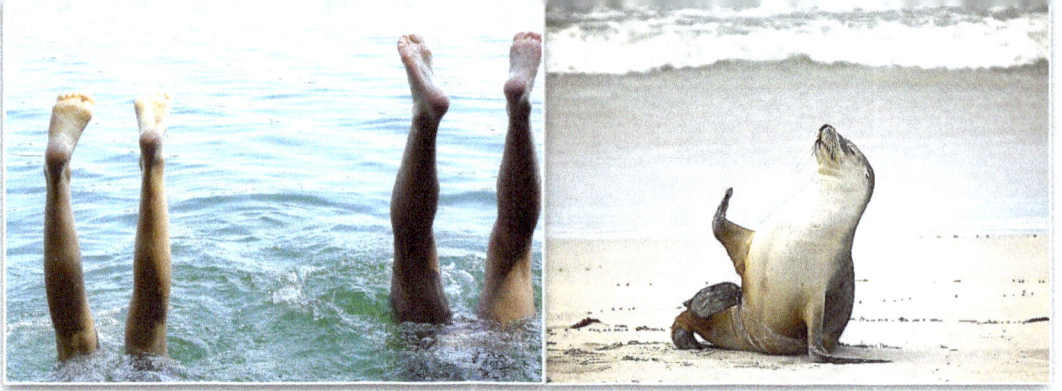

Have the sense that the cord is gliding through water, because it is. Differentiate between internal and external, superior or inferior pulls on the cord. Move your head slightly in each direction to see if that clarifies the source or action of the pull if there is one. If you even feel a little compression around your sacrum or low back, lift your rib cage slightly with your hands, extend your chin out and up slightly, and bend your knees a little more, letting your sacrum fall free. Avoid compressing the spine with any exercise you may enter into. Extend out and away from each vertebrae, giving each disc as much space as you can.

When you feel that you've been able to communicate with each area we've contacted, and have listened and responded to the feedback from your body, release your hands. Begin the arch and curl again, remembering to lift and 'separate' the spine in both directions; while you flex as well as when you arch. This time when you flex, feel up through your neck into the tissue on top of, and the membranes beneath your skull. Check for any imbalance in levels of pull or tension, then take a deep breath and hold it. Wait for the body to respond, then let the breath go and hold the exhalation.

Wait for the additional release and come up slowly. Continue coming up into the arch, this time lifting your chest and head, chin out slightly, knees back or bent, whichever is the most comfortable. Feel into the fascia in front of your cervical spine, drop your rib cage and inhale, open and close your mouth and notice what you feel in the deeper cervical regions. Repeat the motion with your shoulders and feet internally rotated, taking a moderate inhale and hold it. While there gently rock your head from side to side, nod up and down and turn your head back and forth like you're saying no a couple of times. Exhale and repeat the same movements while holding the exhalation. Breathe normally and come up.

Come up, and as smoothly and effortlessly and you can, move through a complete extension on inhale, and flexion with exhale a few times. Slow it down and check again for how smooth it is. If you like, try combining feet internally rotated on flexion, and externally on extension. My body prefers the feet internally rotated for both as it feels more open in the hip and sacroiliac joints that way. When you come back to center this time, give space for whatever your body feels like in response to the recent action, as it helps to integrate the changes that have taken place

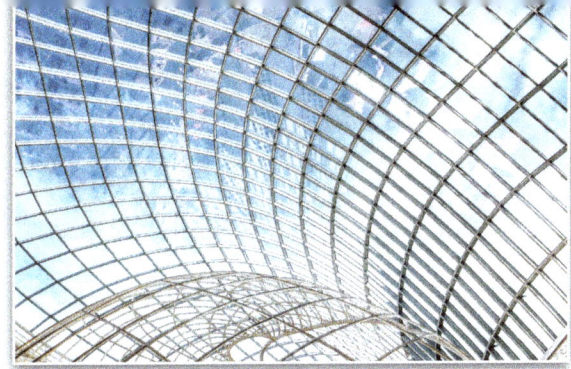

throughout the core. Walk around a bit to further integrate the recent reeducation. Find your own rhythm, and let your body find its own renewed style of moving. It might be better to take a seat for the next piece of reorganization and to allow the legs to rest. You can also sense the subtleties of what's next more easily without feedback from the legs.

Don't worry if you can't sense everything at first. As the soma awakens, it will give you more and more feedback. It may come quickly or gradually, but you will notice it being a little more vibrant each time. Once the physical structures are freer, more balanced, enlivened and talking to one another as their interconnected nature intended, our physiology will also come into more harmony. This usually leads to a better mood, uplifted emotional state, and a clearer mind. When there's less neurological noise and mental chatter in the system, there's more space and calm with which to deepen the inquiry into the more subtle aspects of the soma. That being said, people are different, so it's best not to lay out an expectation.

There are some who are by nature living in the more 'feeling' zone, and those who don't live that way in their senses. You will reap the benefits of tuning in and turning your intention and attention in these areas whether or not you receive immediate feedback from your body, especially for the first few times. As you continue to tune in, your perceptual skills will increase, just like anything you practice. It's a good idea in any case to return to those areas that have proven to be a little sticky, stiff, sore, or resistant to moving. Vary the movement, combination or pairing; the angles you use and the positions you choose. Keep going until you find the sweet spot for those problem areas to the degree that it finds balance and lets go. Make a commitment to keep track of things while they're minor issues.

Now that both the core and extremities are balanced and integrated, let's move inside of the senses themselves. First, tune into your eyes and allow yourself to notice the feeling of the skin of your eyelids, and blink a couple of times so that they stand out a little more in your perception. Then, notice the fluid sensation over your eyes that allow the lids to slide easily across the conjunctiva (the eyeball). Get a sense of the buoyancy of the entire eyeball as well as the shape of it. Notice the different structures in the eye like the cornea, iris, lens, and pupil front and center, then follow the retina around to the back of the eye.

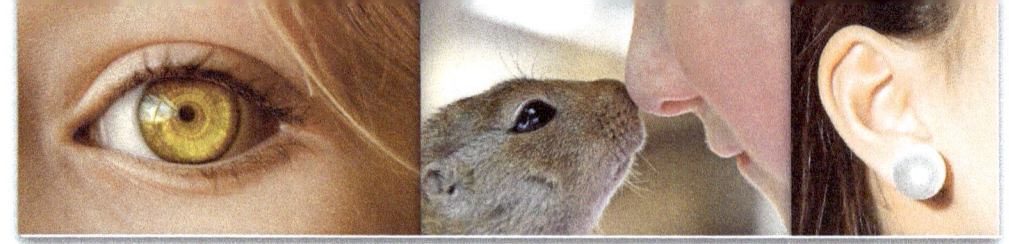

Squeeze them gently so that you can feel the shape and consistency more fully, getting a clearer sense of the vitreous body internally. Move them in each direction just a little distance so you can feel the sense of the small muscles in action. Your body will be tracking with you, so the clearer the identification of landmarks the better. You may notice colors are brighter after! Next, bring your awareness to your nostrils and move them slightly to make them easier to locate with your felt sense. Feel into the bridge of your nose and notice any sensations; contrast from side to side. Then go inside of the nostrils and get a sense of the mucous lining. Feel your breath going inside to get a sense of the surface of the lining and what those surfaces feel like.

Notice if there's a smell to the air that you're breathing, and what it may feel like as it moves across the tiny hairs inside. Feel for the temperature and for how far you can track the sensations into the trachea as well. Do you notice any movement in your neck when the breath enters that area of its path? Try sensing the cavity (the space) in your sinuses. For those of you who know how to wiggle your ears without moving them, do that now and feel where they are on your head. Then feel their connection to your face, jaw, and scalp. Sense the outer helix—the folded edge of the ear above the lobe—and the inner, flatter scapha in front of the canal.

If you wear earrings, can you sense them? Travel locally with your awareness into the canal with the global awareness still on the rest of your body. Take your attention into the inner ear and pause for a few seconds contemplating the structures that enable hearing to happen, like you're listening to what enables us to hear. Make note of anything you do hear, even in the slightest way internally. It may be a high-pitched sound, or a low hum or tiny pulsations or a systemic sound you don't have words for. Next, turn your local attention towards your lips and again, move them if you don't feel anything specific. Get a sense of their edges, the shape and texture.

Move inside your mouth with your awareness and take in the sensations of your tongue, your gums and your teeth, as well as the mandible, the jawbone. Continue to the roof of your mouth and down the back of your throat, including the felt sense of your tonsils if you still have them. Receive any input the deeper structures that surround the esophagus and trachea have to share with you. Wait for the feedback from your brain as to the levels of tension or ease there. Swallow a couple of times and notice if there is a pull to one side. Revisit those muscles if there is. Connect the deeper throat region with your inner ear using your awareness, then include

Sternocleidomastoid muscle (anterior)

the back of your tongue. Your stomach may light up with your attention there and notice the path in between the tongue, and stomach as well, including the lower esophageal or cardiac sphincter. The vagus nerve runs right through this area of the esophagus, so check to see if you notice a little variance in the sensation that distinguishes the lining of the esophagus with a thin, buzzy nerve sensation. If you do, place your palm gently on the buzzy area and wait for the sense of an energetic discharge leaving the area, or a relieving calm entering the area.

Track that sensation back to the sternocleidomastoid muscle as it runs from behind the ear down behind the collar bone onto the first rib and sternum. Notice if there's a matching sensation for the vagus nerve there. Tuning into the nervous system may stimulate an awakening in this nerve which touches the heart, the celiac plexus, the intestines, and more with a type of sparkly, sensation that you now may become aware of. Then, imagine each nerve as part of energetic and blood pathways, which they are. There is a major lymphatic pathway ascending up the core, along with the Conception Vessel, the aorta, and the Primo Vascular vessels surrounding nerves and blood vessels.

Place a finger in your navel along with one in the center of your sternum and feel for an organizational response. You may also notice a Universal rhythm as it lightly rocks back and forth. That rhythm, in and of itself, is calming. Arch and curl a few times to revisit and reintroduce the clarity, fluidity, and spaciousness in the core. Maintain opened senses as you move and allow that balance in the core to permeate the extremities. Have the sense that your brain is floating freely as you move your spine and cord in flexion and extension. Now come back to center in balanced, open, integrated sitting, with blended awareness within and without.

Turn your global awareness to include the force of gravity, however it reveals itself to your perception just now. Realize that there is an upward flowing energy that counterbalances gravity and let them recognize and equalize one another. You may feel like you no longer need to breathe in this type of balance, like the life force and gravitational force are in such equilibrium that you are being breathed. Last, tune into the space in which all of this is being perceived, let that permeate and further enliven and reorganize what and how you are perceiving and rest there. At some later point, go into large movements that may reveal what is left to open using tiny perceptions and tiny adjustments.

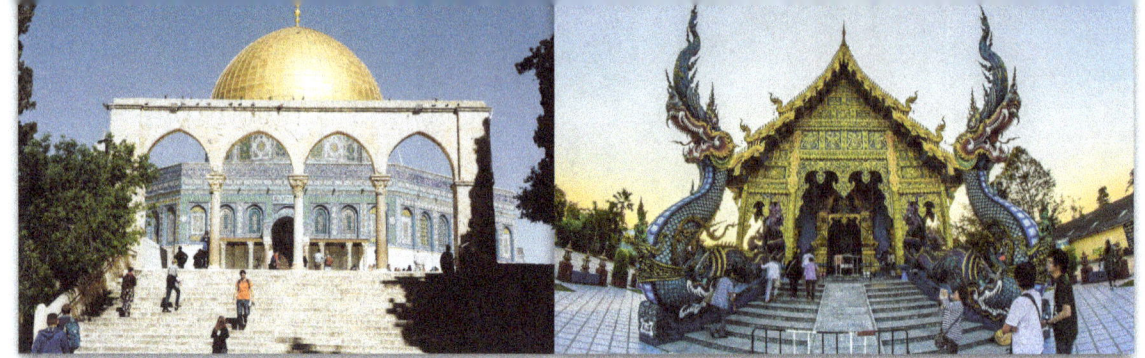

## Healing the last percentages

Healing all the way is a complex process that is likely the most rewarding process you will come into in your life. It transforms the quality of every waking moment and continually opens new vistas that are as awe-inspiring and wonder-filled, as they are in-sight full and deepening. The beauty of it is that whatever it is you're healing from, however long or short it's been with you, the elevation and transfiguration of every experience you'll have afterwards will be touched and infused with the vibrancy inherent in what you've dared to open up. Remember that from this point of view, it's all about the free movement of all systems, from the tiniest to the largest, to optimize all levels of information exchange.

Whether the releases fill you with energies that have been locked away, or empty you of tensions that leave you spacious and content, or both, the explorations will be fulfilling. From the somatic perspective, becoming aware and fully functional is becoming healed. We're not looking for a type of 'perfection' but for an open, sensitive soma that is able to use its intelligence freely, resulting in a health and well-being that is palpably 'unsensational'. From my perspective, there was another driving force alongside of this healthy condition that involved a quest set in motion decades ago. That quest was to see if it was possible to understand the mechanisms of our multi-dimensionality nature. There was this inkling that the entire continuum, from the formless into the form, influenced health, healing, and well-being. I wanted to find out how the integration of Spirit and form did that.

Although there are many subtle systems that influence each another and our body in some way, as mentioned earlier, I only speak here about the ones that were becoming more obvious to me; that were tangible and could be experienced on some level. It would be time well spent for you to discover which ones call to you and echo in your systems. Which ones want to play a more conscious part in your journey of revelation? Meditation is more of a mental state that can access the subtle mental body beyond where the brain resides. We now know that meditation is a very powerful influencer of health. In addition, the concentration it promotes can promote a clear focus for the body that might otherwise be distracted by following the ordinary cascade of thoughts that may not be useful for homeostasis.

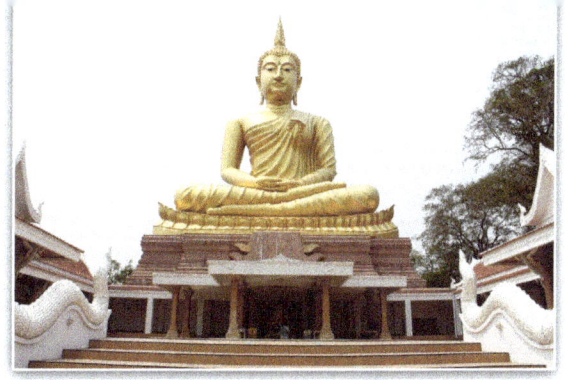

Thought processes can activate all sorts of tension throughout the body. I spoke earlier of states of no-mind that work as a most wonderful frame of reference for the nervous system and brain to organize around. It frees them up to mobilize resources for healing. Concentrating on one object, like the breath, or something that is sacred to you in your heart or in the center of your forehead can also be really beneficial as a frame of reference, as long as the concentrating is relaxed. It's also helpful to perceive of your soma as sacred, because its origins as well as what sustains life is sacred.

Some of the states that are found in the heart or in other states of consciousness produce a type of coherence for the entire system that is also very nourishing and balancing. This coherence acts as a form of communication for every system. Recitation of mantras or reciting prayers, or the higher values of good wishes for kindness, love, compassion, forgiveness, gratitude, peace, and harmony are heard and responded to by the Higher Power. It also invokes a type of coherence into the field. Mother Nature is an expression of the Higher Power. Spending time in her presence offers a coherence that is already realized as balancing and calming to most people. She offers many gifts as foods, natural remedies and frequencies.

By the time the ball strike to the head happened in October, I was well on my way in the research of the properties of essential oils. As I placed them in order on a shelf in my kitchen, I could see the radiance emanating from them, like the liquid light spoken about in our cerebral spinal fluid by Cranial Sacral Pioneers. I decided to develop blends that protect the nerve cells from plaque, from oxidation, from inflammation, from stress chemistry, and that stimulate the production of neurotransmitters and biochemicals that are helpful for cognitive function. I have created inhalers filled with different blends knowing they will touch the olfactory nerve and go straight into the brain. There are also properties in certain oils that either bind to CB1/CB2 receptors, or that stimulate the production of endogenous cannabinoids.

These molecules have properties that allow them to function as cannabinoids, such as beta-caryophyllene and anandamide, meaning that they are messengers that help regulate homeostasis. There are also oils with properties that help release trauma. I've used these oils on a daily basis in inhalers and diffusers, along

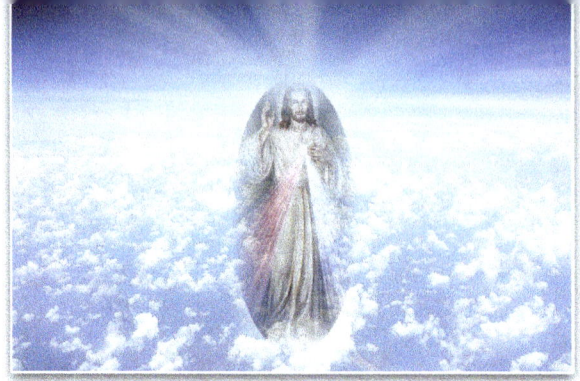

with new forms of brain nutrition such as Brahmi, Cordyceps and Lion's Mane. Knowing that inflammation is the substrate of cell death in the nervous system, I spent more time supporting and detoxing the liver, in addition to using more antioxidant juices like pomegranate and Noni.

I explored many ways of working with the eyes and pairing them with the brain. At times I attempted to sense the optic chiasm, the pulvinar at the back of the thalamus, claustrum, as I paired them with the eyes. What was the most interesting was by settling the agitation in descending pathways as they exited the sensorimotor cortex, in addition to settling other visual regions in the midbrain. Opening up restrictions in the superior vena cava, the jugular, and entry into the atrium of the heart has been incredibly helpful. I spent more time on the lymph and exit points of the meridians in the arms, as congestion there was limiting range of motion in my shoulders and retaining emotional content.

All of these have been significant in their ability to clear both subtle and grosser systems, and have paved the way for enhanced communication between them, as well as in my ability to share a common vocabulary with them. The Grace and presence of those teachers and spiritual masters I've met and been able to contact in Consciousness was just as important as any supplement, exercise, or dietary changes that were made. Whatever Higher Power or angel you relate to, including your own soul will also be ever present to assist in your healing intentions. It seemed that each layer or dimension was part of the entire fabric of my being. Nourishing the attention and awareness of one layer can nourish them all when they are aligned and integrated.

Each contributed to the ability to heal all the way because in order for the integration to be all-inclusive, all that we are needs to be awakened as much as possible and participating in the conversation. Obstructions or adhesions that contribute to inaccurate or distorted information can happen and become stored in forms as subtle as energy, thought, attitude, fluids, cells of organs or nerves, fascia, and even bone. As long as they remain subconscious, they will have an effect that interferes with any healing process that can shorten lifespans and decrease the quality of the days we do live in. It can become surviving instead of

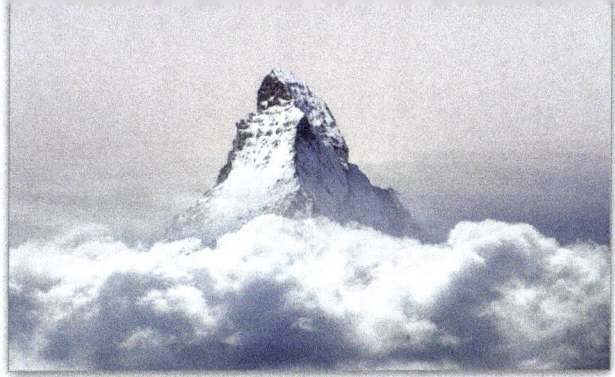

thriving. Consciously bringing life and space into these areas is as transformative as it is informative. Very often, the tiniest inquiry has the most global effect.

Going for the tiny explorations in any arena you can learn to discern will uncover more and more potential for deeper freedom. I make it a point to do a scan every evening before bed, and every morning before getting out of bed. Today I had the most amazing response imaginable just by making the tiniest of movements with each finger. The response was all over my body and particularly reflected back into the brachial plexus at the base of the neck in a relieving way. Like the eyes, the hands are connected to everything we do, and have quite a bit of real estate in the brain. The location on the homunculus for the hands and fingers happens to be just where I banged my head on the freezer door, and I can see how they can also help to relieve noise in the CNS related to tinnitus.

My brain was incredibly quiet after this. I may also begin releasing my neck using my fingers! I will make this a regular practice, along with mini-movements of my toes, as that effort this morning also released my hips. Changes are happening all the time, so I can't assume that the body's status the day before will be the same the next day. Checking in regularly affords a new opportunity to see how well your system is adapting to your activities. Increasing fluency and wakefulness in the body's sensorial vocabularies increases the probability that it will be able to handle almost anything with ease, as long as you continue to listen. Awakening and exploring all of these layers and minuscule places in my own system has helped to uncover many of the reasons for the injuries happening in the first place, and will likely prevent that form of creating lessons in the future.

Once the clouds over the subtle bodies and energetic systems are removed, the beauty and bounty afforded by increasing awareness transmit the type of liberation that your soul is made of. It's like coming home to a place that is irreplaceable. Experiencing the multitude of injuries brought something into my life that could never have unfolded the same way without them. At this point I feel like I'm at a modest 98% healed, and although I will continue to grow and evolve in what self-sensing unveils and eagerly await what could be revealed if that 2% finds a reason to show a symptom. And honestly, I'm not wanting to attract that mechanism in the Universe that behaves sometimes as the Trickster who jumps in to test your thesis!

My little scars remind me to check in regularly and take care. They remind me to look there first if something feels a little off. They are a source of motivation and leave me a place to aspire to for greater understanding and reeducation. For example, while contemplating the field of the heart the other day, I followed it out to its edges and contacted the Heart of the Whole, somehow already present and listening to my exploration. How could it be otherwise, when the exploration is happening within its own field? However, the intent of this particular exploration opened up a response in a new way - and the response was infinite love. It made me wonder what would need to happen in a somatic exploration for each person to realize that an infinite amount of love was nearer than their own breath?

This particular time I was feeling into the field around the brain, and the field around the heart and belly brain, and fortuitously discovered the mechanism of their interconnection on an energy level, using biophotons. As I moved out to the edges of the electromagnetic field of the heart, beyond the activity of the systems interacting with one another, was the Intelligence and love of the Whole as consciousness. Because I was feeling into these spaces with my heart, the Whole responded with its Heart. I've seen this before, whereby Existence responds according to the question and to how you're asking it.

Although all of this may seem like a lot to go through at first, the rewards are not like having your favorite meal, or visiting a gorgeous island for vacation. Those things are over pretty quick. This process is a living one that continues to exist as long as you do. Realizing that every living thing we're in the presence of also has a presence and intelligence full of information to share is mind-boggling. When you also learn the languages it communicates with, it is life altering. Even after you've healed your stress, pain, heart, mind, energy and spirit, the possibilities of what can still be learned are endless. Your ability to function well in everyday life will still always be improved with self-sensing and self-regulation, but just remember that there's something larger that is also sensing and regulating you.

Awareness is the key that unlocks every door within. Awareness is a 'field' that is more subtle than energetic systems, which enables them to be perceived. Awareness itself is devoid of pain, disease, dysfunction or any of the issues of the body/mind. When tuning into Awareness—that which enables you to pay attention to anything—your system can organize around that empty quality of consciousness and use it to help the healing process. Awareness can become shrouded by the parts of us that are unconscious and subject to the forces activated in the hindbrain, and by our attention resting in mental or emotional states, rather than in the space that is liberated from them.

That said, it's natural for the attention to travel to whatever pain or stress that presents in front of us. That's the body's language for an area that needs more attention to fully heal back into the larger body, and the body's larger field. Just know that you as the fulcrum can return to the empty, neutral space of being awareness itself. I can attest to the fact that every year, each exploration of every injury sends me more deeply into a level of healing I'd never have known was possible. That may have even been their purpose. The infinite intelligence that we are surrounded by always has more to reveal to us.

The more that we are inspired to awaken to all of what we are, and listen to more of these intricate forms of intelligence, the closer we will be to discovering our infinite potential. Our bodies are different every single millisecond, as are the experiences we are in front of, as well as our options of how to interact with them. That inquiry enlivens and enriches the very fabric that we live and breathe through, for which you are likely going to feel eternal gratitude in such a way that you'll feel inspired to share it, as countless people already have done. What better gift to share than peace and freedom?

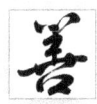

*"Tis the mortar in the Space between the bricks that holds the structure together."*

*~ Dr. William Sutherland*

*"You can actually feel something other in the laws (of linear cause and effect) as you witness them. Let's ponder this by sensation as we live and treat; let's look again for a greater geometry than cause and effect."*

*~ Dr. James Jealous*

*"...Each of us contains everything that ever was or will be, within ourselves. We have only to learn... how to open to this omniscient area within us to obtain this information."*

*~ Swami Rudrananda*

*"The mind is asked to find the connection between the physical and the spiritual"*

*~ Dr. A.T. Still*

# About the Author

Suresha has lived a lifetime of curiosity and fascination about the human condition and how to possibly improve, if not uplift the experiences and challenges attached to being born. She began studying Sociology at Kentucky State University, then switched majors to Elementary and Special Education when she transferred to Kent State University in 1970. After earning a Bachelor of Science Degree, she went on to earn M.S. and Ed.S. degrees in School Psychology, with a Specialty in Prevention and Systems Intervention.

After a few years of practicing in her fields of study including the psychology of change, she saw that many of the learning problems in children were related to neurological, physiological, and emotional issues. Her studies then extended to energetic systems like Shiatsu and Polarity, Breath Therapy, Hypnotherapy, Anatomy, Physiology, the musculoskeletal system, Visceral Manipulation (internal organ treatment), Brain Classes, the Lymphatic System, Hanna Somatic Education, a diploma in Osteopathy, a Biodynamic Cranial Sacral Therapy Training, and a few other modalities. Along the way, she'd been a martial artist in Isshin Ryu karate, along with Dwa Shaan, and various forms of Chi Kung.

She danced and played a variety of sports for her entire life, and began a Spiritual focus in 1978, whereby she studied with a variety of teachers and a few Spiritual Masters. She also wrote for a newspaper for three years, worked for a Public Relations firm as an interviewer and writer, and wrote several books. "Remember the Wisdom that Progress Forgot - Sharing the Gems of our Ancestors" took 15 years to complete as a tribute to her ancestry. The first three volumes in the Somatic Intelligence series were written for students of the NeuroSomatic Integration work she developed. Somatic Intelligence Volume 4 was entitled, "What your Body is Dying for You to Know," Volume 5 is, "The Conversation Every Body Wants to Have with You," and Volume 6 is, "Opposing Gravity - How to Recognize and Heal from Head Injuries."

She worked many years for chiropractors, Wellness Centers, and a Sports Medicine clinic until 1992, when she founded the Marin Center for Somatic Integration. Suresha taught Somatics, along with various aspects of NeuroMuscular Reeducation for 25 years. She became the owner and CEO of Shibui Gardens Spa in 2005, where she continues her practice supporting the community in a variety of methods that help them to regain or retain health and well-being. Her vision is to inspire the desire to heal into wholeness.

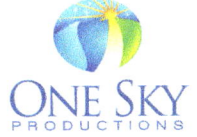

www.ingramcontent.com/pod-product-compliance
Lightning Source LLC
Chambersburg PA
CBHW060424010526
44118CB00017B/2343